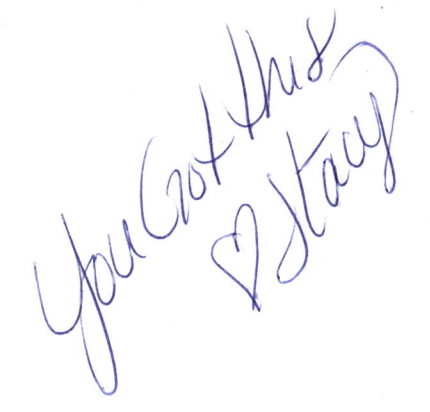

KICKING ANXIETY IN THE ASS
...A LITTLE AT A TIME

THIS IS MORE THAN JUST A BOOK

This book is full of resources and links that are best accessed online. Anywhere you see <u>text that looks like this</u> know that there is corresponding content online.

Go to <u>http://kickinganxietybook.com/links</u> or scan the QR code below to get free access to an interactive PDF.

Copyright © 2020 by Stacy Tiegs

all rights reserved. No part of this book may be reproduced or used in any manner without written permission of the copyright owner except for the use of quotations in a book review.

Paperback ISBN: 978-1-7352767-0-0

Digital ISBN: 978-1-7352767-1-7

DEDICATION

I'm dedicating this book to my youngest daughter, Emily. I've never been more proud of how far she has come. She has such a big heart, and I'm so grateful she is now helping others because of what she learned through her past.

She has taught me many things.

We love you, Emmerz.

Stacy Tiegs

CONTENTS

PART 1: THE STORY 6

Walking on Eggshells 7

The Roller Coaster from Hell 9

The Toll of Social Stigma 11

Anything but Normal 12

Credit Cards & Pain Clinics 15

Miracles Really Do Happen 18

An Epidemic 20

Formation of Our Identity 22

Goodbye Coffee Creamer 23

Breaking Free 26

Kicking Its Ass 29

PART 2: THE HOW 32

The Crisis in Our Cells 33

The Toxic Overload 34

Your Skin Eats Everything 39

Could a deficiency be the problem? 44

The Gut-Brain Connection 44

Parasites: Ever thought you could have these? 48

We Really ARE What We Eat 49

It all starts in the morning 61

School Lunches 63

Fast Food 64

PART 3: WHERE DO I START? 66

    Food Choices to Consider..67

    Nutritional Supplementation 90

    Managing - Action Items..97

    Solving the Puzzle of anxiety...108

PERSONAL REFLECTION 110
EPILOGUE 111
MY FAVORITE RESOURCES... 114
CONTACT ME 117
ACCOLADES.. 118
ABOUT THE AUTHOR 120
ENDNOTES.. 121

PART 1: THE STORY

"The only way for a woman, as for a man, to truly find herself, to know herself as a person, is by creative work of her own. There is no other way."

-Betty Friedan

I finally decided I can no longer stay silent.

I wish I could go back in time and share this knowledge and mental strategy to help my Emily and myself years ago. What I learned throughout this journey was to keep an open mind and not be in such a hurry to fix things. We learned not to just cover our issues with band-aids, but instead to take time to ask questions and seek answers. The old me was a really busy mom who wanted the quickest and cheapest way to skid through life, especially when it came to our health. The new me has learned a better way, and through our story and this guide, I hope to help you find your 'better way' too.

It's all about the little things and knowing the little things add up to the big things. It's not about blaming yourself for a past you can no longer control, but how you can start today to make positive change happen in your daily life. It's not about just one thing that's the problem. It's about slowly peeling back the layers to unveil the root causes of the real issue. Don't do what I did either. Don't skip through the story pages to just find bullet points and do what looks easy for you to do. The meat and potatoes of this book is in Part 2 and 3, but you need to understand Part 1 - the WHY. Anxiety, in my opinion, is like a puzzle, and you need to take the time to fit in each piece to see the whole picture.

You can choose the "just getting by" attitude, or you can choose to work hard and dig to find the root cause. Take the time to empower yourself and self-educate. Let this book be your self education. Part 2 and 3 are a lifestyle guide filled with many ways to start looking at new choices and how you can slowly create new habits. Everyone can start by doing something small today. If you or anyone you know is struggling with anxiety or depression, I know this book will help you kick it in the ass - a little at a time.

WALKING ON EGGSHELLS

I'll never forget that morning. What I thought was going to be a typical morning, a morning of coffee and flipping through news channels, ended up taking a drastic turn in the opposite direction. That idyllic image is nothing close to what I was about to endure. I woke up to blood-curdling screams in my kitchen the likes of which I have never heard before. Loud, pitchy outbursts of madness like the girl in the Exorcist movie. I literally thought someone was dying.

I quickly threw on my robe and ran out into the kitchen, where I saw my 16-year-old daughter at the top of the stairs screaming her lungs out. I didn't even recognize her facial expressions through the red face and tears of rage. My thoughts raced: "Is this really happening? Is this really my child right now? How can I fix this?" I immediately looked around for blood, gashes or severed limbs....and I saw nothing of the sort.

As I got closer, I hysterically asked her, "What is wrong???" and at the top of her lungs she screamed,

"MY CAR WON'T START."

That's it? Her car wouldn't start? As I looked at my panic-stricken daughter, all I wanted to say was, "Are you for real?"

We had no idea where these outbursts came from. My husband, Tom, and I wondered if she was on some kind of hallucinogenic drugs. Or maybe it was a side effect from her anxiety medications or imbalanced hormones from her period; who really knew? After experiencing that outburst on the stairs, I knew there was something more we needed to look into. Something was terribly wrong and I needed to fix it. I just didn't know how.

I remember when Emily was really little she hated socks. They irritated her and she stomped her feet in agitation all the time. I absolutely dreaded the fight every morning we needed to put a pair of socks on. Most days she went without! Even on the way to the school bus stop, I'd watch her through the window as she stomped her feet with her face clenched in rage the whole way there. We must have spent thousands of dollars on shoes hoping they would make her socks more tolerable.

We started noticing she was irritated at other things too. Like if someone in the room was chewing, or if the music or TV was too loud for her liking. Or when it was really quiet in the house and she could hear her sister breathing through her nose. Little things like this would trigger her to instantly get up from the table, push her fingers into her jaw and walk straight to her room. We rarely ate at the table as a family for this reason.

Being busy parents, we would just say, "That's our Emily". We were all walking on eggshells. But she was our last child; whatever Emily wanted, we gave it to her. My son actually called her "The Chosen One". Nobody really wanted to deal with her emotions. Nobody ever gave much thought to why this was happening; and nobody knew where it came from.

THE ROLLER COASTER FROM HELL

Emily had always been quiet and introverted, but when she really started tuning us out and her grades started to drop, I knew there was a bigger issue. We watched her slowly isolate herself and completely withdraw from social activities. We tried a few support groups that were totally ineffective. Attending groups may have made us a little more aware of our issues as parents, but we honestly didn't connect with other families that well. Being in a large circle talking about our problems was not giving us the answers we sought.

We were busy; not neglectful by any means, but you know, we were just like any other mother and father. We were raising children the best we knew how while working full time to support our family. We worked to demonstrate hard work and good ethics to our kids, and for the most part, they respected both of us. So from the very beginning, we often wondered what Emily could possibly have to be depressed about. As the months continued, there was no denying she needed help.

As Emily entered the 7th grade, we took her in for a mental check-up at the clinic. That led to the diagnosis of anxiety and depression, and Emily was on a daily medication at the age of thirteen.

A few months after she started the medications, her jaw problems began to worsen. I took her to a specialist, and he told me he had never seen a girl her age with such tight jaw muscles. She had an extreme case of TMJ. That made my heart break. WHY was my sweet girl clenching so badly? As the months rolled on, we booked appointments with more specialists, endured constant hours of electric stimulation and chiropractic care, and tried every mouth appliance known to mankind. We had no idea the muscle pain could also be tied to emotions of anxiety and depression. We spent thousands of dollars in vain researching the symptom, but failed to seek the root cause.

It felt as though we were on a roller coaster ride from hell. Some days weren't so bad. But some days, Emily didn't come home from school. Now at 16, she was ignoring all the rules and doing what she wanted when she wanted. Emily even threw parties when Tom and I would leave for the weekend. We would come home and find evidence of some serious ragers. Having an in-ground pool made it a fun place for everyone - especially when the parents are gone. The potential liability we could have been responsible for was too awful to even think about. When the neighbors told me there were cars coming in and out, kids blaring music (probably drinking), and kids jumping from our roof down into the pool, I really was starting to wonder where we went wrong. I was living a parent's nightmare.

How had we allowed the situation to get this bad? We tried many common forms of discipline. Grounding her never really worked, nor did taking away her phone. In fact, pretty much everything we tried only seemed to make things worse. The harsh reality was that we were just busy, young and naive parents who didn't even realize there was a problem until Emily was out of control.

THE TOLL OF SOCIAL STIGMA

In her junior year, Emily chose an alternative learning center instead of high school. This is the type of school where the class sizes were small and manageable and had more individualized learning. The smaller environment made it somewhat easier for Emily to control her anxiety. The teachers were excellent, but deep down I was devastated that my baby girl wouldn't graduate with all the "normal" kids. She would get her diploma, but in a different way.

I struggled with the stigma over my failures with my daughter. What would all my friends say? What kind of mom am I? I'm saddened to say we made decisions for our daughter out of fear of what others would think. I hate how society can manipulate us and how we inadvertently let it decide how we live our lives. I let others think for me because I never felt smart enough or equipped to handle the really tough situations. The herd was comforting, and I was like a sheep and just followed along. I never asked any questions. Instead, I conformed to what everyone else was doing. It's what I was used to. It was easy.

Admittedly, our communication wasn't always the best either. We may have avoided confrontations in favor of hoping things would just somehow work themselves out. If I couldn't communicate with Emily verbally, we just covered it up with mall and shopping therapy. I thought having clothes from Abercrombie & Fitch and Hollister would make her happy. But that was not the answer. What was so awful to cause this kind of depression? Was it her friends and relationships? Were we not spending enough time with her? Were we not nurturing enough? Or could it be the side effects from a new anxiety med she was taking? We tried about eight different medications over the years, and surprisingly enough—she was still a mess. Why was she still not happy?

She considered online school, but it wasn't a good fit for her. I respected her for researching options and not giving up. I had no choice but to trust her decision to attend the learning center and believe it would be better than what she was going through in high school. In truth, I was so proud of her then for making an effort to advocate for herself, and I still am.

Prior to Emily's setbacks, I knew nothing about anxiety and depression. I had no idea how it could tear a person apart, let alone an entire family. I was too busy being busy. Most of the time, I felt totally helpless and beat myself up with guilt for not seeing the signs sooner. Here's the biggest lesson I learned: Get in touch with your kids RIGHT NOW. Ask questions and spend quality time with them. It's never too late. Don't dismiss any odd behavior, and don't think it will work itself out on its own. Trust me. I found out a few years later that at one point Emily considered taking her own life. I will forever be grateful she never followed through.

ANYTHING BUT NORMAL

The funny thing about life is that it doesn't just stop when you're stressed to the gills. While our family endured what we thought were "normal teenage issues", other things were about to change. And I mean really change.

While teenage dramas were in full swing, Tom was running his own heating and plumbing business. He was a master at being a provider for our family. He even hired me as his secretary. I helped with bookkeeping, paying the bills, and filing. I ordered all the uniforms for employees, planned annual vacations for our team, and kept the office quite clean. I enjoyed the flexibility the job provided, but the downfall was when you work for your husband, there is no room for advancement or promotion. Trust me when I say, there is little glamour in the title of "Husband's Secretary." Think about it: Could you work side-by-side with your husband? Every day? Eat, sleep and work together for eight years? I definitely didn't plan for those ups and downs.

My husband has a knack for planning and he's very smart when it comes to the economy and what's going on. In 2008, he foresaw the new construction business coming to a halt. This was when he told me that I needed to get a "real job". I'll never forget sitting in his office trying to absorb those words. At first I was a little upset he was telling me to look for work. I had no idea where I could work that would offer the same flexibility. Working for him gave me more time with the kids, which was important because he was never home. When he told me I had to start bringing in some income, I instantly felt the freedom of my Queen of Sheba life leaving my existence in one breath.

And so my job search began. I knew right away that I was not cut out for your typical 9-5 job, and I needed more flexibility than the traditional job would allow. I knew I would not give my blood, sweat and tears to build someone else's dream. I did that for almost ten years before my husband became self employed. I knew I was meant to find something more exciting; something more - fun.

Then one day my amazing sister, Carrie Green, showed me a few pieces of jewelry she was making for some friends. They were beautiful and I was intrigued, so I asked her to teach me how to make a few pieces. Over the next few months, Carrie and I made so much jewelry, my husband suggested we try to sell some of it. The next thing I knew, I was opening my own brick-and-mortar boutique store and filling it up with things to sell. And when I say filling it up, I was f-i-l-l-i-n-g i-t u-p.

This is when the debt really kicked into high gear.

Then - I had an idea. As I was knee deep in thousands of beads and tools, why not teach other people to make jewelry too? So on top of running the boutique, I taught women and children how to make jewelry. There was no better way to do that than during a party. So that led to hosting children's birthday parties and ladies-night-outs. Oh, were those fun. We were booked solid; sometimes doing ten parties in one weekend.

I rented two spaces at one point; one for kids and the other with the Bead Bar for the ladies. Women would come sit up at the Bead Bar and create some pretty unique things. I loved everything about it. Another reason why I loved doing the parties was because I didn't have to worry about finding lunch or dinner. I never planned ahead, and this was just so convenient. I ate with everyone and would eat whatever they brought in. Pizza, cake, cupcakes, Culvers ice cream, candy bags...I was in Heaven!

Entertaining was fun, and I love to socialize. People even came back again and again to create more, and kids came back year after year to have their birthday party at my store. That right there lit up my world. I was passionate about what I was doing and how I could make those kids feel energized and happy. All the smiles, all the laughter, all the whipped cream we sprayed in their faces - I made sure every child's birthday was one to remember.

I had finally found my dream job and I dove in head first. But even though I loved what I was doing, I was still drowning in debt. There was a shit storm brewing, people. An out-of-control tornado was on its way.

CREDIT CARDS & PAIN CLINICS

I loved spending money. I was careless, and I didn't know what a budget was or how to manage employees, much less how to make a profit. There were no 3-5 year plans or any written goals. I had absolutely no structure for running my business. I dabbled in a little coaching and even cashed in an IRA to pay for it, but I was just too disorganized and made a myriad of foolish decisions. I just thank GOD for those who stuck with me when I didn't have a clue.

When I told my husband I was going to make millions opening this store, he believed and trusted me. But I didn't have a plan. I thought I could handle it after seeing how my husband ran his business, but I quickly learned that typing up bids and paying bills was completely different than running a full-blown business. I remember always being nervous to hire someone, as I really wasn't sure how I could pay them. Like, no joke. This is when those credit cards sure came in handy.

At one point, I had five maxed-out credit cards with a lot of old debt. I let this eat me up for years. My store had three locations during that time period, and that always seemed to cost me more with signs, graphics and advertising. I remember one time my husband came to my office and saw a credit card bill for $15,000 lying on my desk. I was sweating bullets. I could literally feel my heart pounding out of my chest and it felt like I was going to die. Tom HATED debt and always made sure we didn't have any personal debt of our own.

Right after we got married, he paid off all of my credit cards and said there would be no more. "If you can't pay for something in full, then you can't afford it," he would say. Well, silly me, I must have forgotten that.

I wasn't sure what to do at that point. He had no idea there were other cards I was hiding; and I hid them well after that. Can you imagine the stress? Can you imagine the anxiety, shame and defeat I felt? I just wanted him to be proud of me for running a store all by myself. I didn't want him to find out how bad it really was and shut my doors down. I had nothing else going for me as far as skills, and I wasn't ready to have my dreams crushed. Not yet.

Here's the kicker though.

I was twice my current body size taking an average ten pills a day for pain, stress, tachycardia, sleep, yeast infections, sinus infections, cold sores, energy and whatever else I could get to instantly fix me. I was losing hair, addicted to sugar and knew nothing about food quality. I ate what I wanted when I wanted, easily opened that second bottle of wine, and didn't have a clue about vitamins or nutrition. Do ya think maybe this played a role in the stress too?

Years prior, I had undergone five hip surgeries, that's when I needed pain meds. I had nine cortisone shots, EKG's, arthrograms, countless MRI's, CT scans, saw multiple ENT specialists, cardiology specialists and endured four heart monitors for heart palpitations. I was also in and out of different pain clinics for a few years. It was so easy to get wrapped up in myself and all this. I actually felt validated having all these things wrong with me. Isn't that crazy? I had great insurance that paid for everything. My co-pay was $10.00, and my refills came quick.

If I had a problem, there was always something quick to fix it. Even in my marriage. Antidepressants were cheaper than leaving, so that was my plan. Oh, you know you've all thought about it once or twice too. But I believed that addressing the real issues would just add more stress, stir the pot, per say, and who had time to deal with emotions or have real conversations about them? It was called a broom and a rug, and we just kept sweeping the shit under it.

> Sometimes I felt if I was less stressed and less of a tornado myself, I wouldn't have been so quick to put Emily on medication. But pills came naturally to me because that's all I knew.

By now, the whole family was on antidepressants, with the exception of my son. On top of antidepressants, my husband was also taking pain meds for his knees. He was almost four sizes larger than he is today because of his poor diet and lack of exercise. He ate fast food frequently along with supersized Cokes on ice; and don't forget the Party Pizzas and Mountain Dew®. We loved all the quick and easy foods that were packaged up for convenience. We never considered what we were actually consuming on a daily basis. And we definitely didn't think twice about the ingredients or how "toxins" could affect us later on.

In my case I was: A toxic, stressed out mom, broke business owner twice my current body size, with a super-sized, medicated family. In reality, we were just getting by day by day numbing ourselves. And I felt like this was normal because everyone else was doing the same thing. Most businesses have debt, most marriages suck, most kids are medicated, and most Americans are overweight - at least that's what I thought.

As I look back on all this, there wasn't one person who asked us what our diet was like. There wasn't one person who asked us about the things we were putting in or on our bodies. No one asked if we had emotional trauma from the past that we were burying alive. Nobody asked where the stress was coming from or why we were all depressed. The easy fix for me was refills, and over time they became a habit.

I believe there is a time and place for medication, but I strongly feel it should only be a short term fix while we figure out a long term solution. If you're okay with what you're currently taking and it's serving you, then by all means give yourself permission to do what feels right for you.

MIRACLES REALLY DO HAPPEN

One day as I was working, a beautiful woman walked into my store. I remember she was holding a little pink bottle of something in her hand. She wore a white coat, and I swear she had a halo over her head just like an angel. Her name was Jewels. I remember that moment clear as day. There was nobody else in the store, and I actually remember being happy I had time to be present with her. She sat up at my Bead Bar and we chatted for a long time, and then she told me about essential oils. These were brand new to me, but she said she taught classes and thought my store would be a perfect place for one. At the time, they looked expensive, so I didn't really take her seriously until I smelled that bottle of Joy™ she was holding. She gave me an experience that day, and I will never forget it.

I enrolled in Young Living in 2012, and this is when I finally learned there was a better way. I listened to Jewels and hosted an oils class in my store, and I had no idea that all of the free education I received that night would change the course of my family's life forever.

From my previous involvement in other network marketing companies, five to be exact, this was a completely different experience. There wasn't anything salesey about it. Not one thing. I was worried about the cost though. I never thought about the "worth" of something, just about the money going out. I thought, "Oh man, if it's natural, it's going to cost me more." That word natural just sounded expensive. But during the class, she shared valid points and hit home with crazy awesome testimonies. All of a sudden the price tag didn't matter. The stories I heard about emotions and how this could help my Emily was all that mattered. How can you put a price tag on that? Jewels knew I had a need, and she offered possible solutions - so I signed up with a kit. Thank God someone opened my mind to something different because God knew I needed a plan. He also knew I needed to become more teachable.

When I first opened this little white box, I really didn't know what I was doing. I remember one night when Emily was sleeping, I loaded the diffuser with Bergamot and placed it as close to her head as possible. As I stood there, I was thinking, "How stupid is this? What is this scented mist really going to do?" I even found myself blowing it in her face! One night, as I was swatting the scented mist towards her nose with my hand, she woke up and told me I was the new psycho snake-oil-mom. But there I was, night after night, bawling my eyes out dripping Valor® on her feet and praying for a miracle.

I'll never forget, one day she was headed out the door for school and she said she didn't have any oils on. I remember someone telling me the importance of being consistent, so I quickly ran and grabbed the Valor® and shook it on her like a priest with holy water as she walked out the door. It probably got in her eyes, and her white shirt looked like she had rolled in a pile of blueberries, but I didn't care. I was determined to help her fix this.

Then, it happened.

Less than a month later, things were different...amazingly different. I started seeing my Emily come back. How could something so simple make such a difference? Was it a placebo effect? If so, I didn't care. I was finally consistent at something, and there was no denying that she was getting better.

In the back of my mind I kept thinking about how many other moms were going through what I was going through. How many other moms had NO flipping idea that with a few small changes, life could be so different. Once I realized and accepted that it wasn't a placebo effect and understood that my daughter was actually improving, I began to really think. And I mean, really think.

A few months later, my Emily was back to normal. After starting our oil journey, incorporating a few small diet changes, and being more open with her in communication, she was the happiest I had seen her in a really long time. Don't get me wrong, there were days when challenges still made themselves known. But after watching my daughter go from the imbalanced and volatile mess that she was, to a pill-free, relatively normal teenager, I began wondering if there was a chance of normalcy for me too.

AN EPIDEMIC

Growing up, I moved twelve times and attended eight different schools. My father was an Air Force recruiter and moving became a normal thing. I never knew how long I would be at a school or where we would live next. Because of all the moving around, I never felt grounded or developed real, solid relationships. I couldn't get involved much in after school activities because we were always on the go. I mentally felt like I could never finish anything.

I barely graduated from high school, and my wall boasted no degrees, certificates or black-framed plaques with my name on them. I wasn't known for being good in academics, sports, music or anything special at all. As an adult, I had to learn how to overcome my feelings of self doubt, insecurity and low self-worth that resulted.

Unfortunately, that pattern repeated with my eldest daughter, Samantha. Samantha had more "perfectionist" tendencies like her father. And like her younger sister, she was on antidepressants for six years because of her insecurities. They numbed and shielded her from dealing with her own limiting beliefs of not being good enough. One example from her time in middle school: Samantha used to set her alarm for 5:00 A.M. every morning to make sure she had enough time to make her hair and makeup perfect. She wanted to fit in so badly with the girls at school, but she never thought she was pretty enough. She constantly compared herself to others to the point where she wouldn't get out of bed, so I would call and tell the school she was sick.

This is an epidemic, and we as parents need to help our kids know that they are good enough and show them positive ways to fill that void sooner rather than later. We can't depend on teachers or friends to provide these lessons for our kids. We have to take a proactive stance and teach them the skills they need to develop a healthy identity.

But before we can truly help them, before we can truly help our children, we have to help ourselves. I wish I had known this sooner. We have to face our own giants and be willing to do the hard work to overcome our own insecurities first.

FORMATION OF OUR IDENTITY

Days of Our Lives used to be one of my favorite TV shows. Everyone loves the drama. Everyone loves the beautiful couples, the romance, the perfect marriage, and of course, the betrayal. That's what I thought life should look like. I watched it for years. Little did I know, it shaped a part of my expectations for my own marriage and relationships in a lot of ways. It set me up for those unmet expectations and I had no idea this was why.

It took me years to realize that the T.V. could actually program our thoughts that would turn into beliefs. The average person watches 35 hours of television every week. What about your children? What are they watching? Are they watching something that adds value to their lives? Something that teaches them life skills? Or are they being modeled with unrealistic expectations?

By the age of ten, a child's beliefs about themselves are already formed based on their perception of what they're seeing on television, along with what parents, grandparents, teachers, friends, and other role-models say or have said about them. I mean, when I was ten years old, I just wanted Gilligan to get off the island. Nowadays, kids are trying to keep up with the Kardashian's.

They don't have the mental capacity to decide for themselves at that age what to believe about who they are.

Growing up, what were your parents or role models telling you about yourself? What were you watching on T.V? What kind of friends did you have? Did someone tell you that you were ugly or fat or embarrass you in front of others? Did someone tell you that you were stupid and would never amount to anything - and then you believed it? Those thoughts run our subconscious mind. Your subconscious is the part of your mind that notices and remembers information when you are not actively trying to do so, and it can influence your behavior even though you may not realize it.

Your subconscious mind never forgets.

I often think of what I could have done differently with Samantha. I never asked her WHY she got up two hours early for school to do her hair. What was she watching on T.V.? What was she believing about herself? I had no idea she was that insecure about her image. I would have told her she was beautiful, perfect and loved for who she is.

Whatever identity you formed about yourself in the past, you have the power to forgive, release it, and like my 4 year old granddaughter says, "Let it go".

GOODBYE COFFEE CREAMER

The year I started Young Living was the year I committed to making even more changes regarding my health and the health of my family. Even though I had no clue what I was doing, I attended a few more classes and educational events. I can't even begin to tell you how many notes I took.

I became a student. I started reading everything I could get my hands on about natural health, essential oils, and why organic matters. This is when I quit drinking the sugar-filled coffees with artificial creamers and started drinking Ningxia Red®. I had no idea how addicted I was to sugar until I stopped consuming it. I was amazed at how much better I felt almost immediately, so I knew that just this small change would keep me going in the right direction.

The more I learned, the more empowered I felt. I also listened to audiobooks and podcasts in the car instead of listening to music. Yeah, at first they were boring, but it's extremely rewarding when you learn from those you want to be like. I love jamming out to music, but I was hungry for more knowledge. Did someone say "free college"?

This was a time of tremendous growth for me. Self development education is exactly what I needed. I got permission to think for myself, and this gave me the confidence to open my eyes to new things.

I also dove head first into learning about functional medicine. Functional medicine focuses on identifying and addressing the root cause of disease or illness. This was something I had never heard of, nor did I have any clue about the concept of getting to the "root" cause of anything. Functional medicine asks why, and I wanted all the answers.

I remained consistent. Consistency always wins. Even if it's a negative habit, over time, consistency will show itself. It's the small changes that lead to the bigger ones.

Vulnerability was the next big piece of the puzzle. I finally allowed myself to let go and open up to others about my shit. That alone saved my life. They say you are the average of the five people you hang around. If you associate with negativity or those who love the drama, you will eventually become the negative and the drama queen. Trust the friends who support you and listen to you. Surround yourself with people who inspire positivity and positive change for your life. Those are the people you get vulnerable with. Those are the people you need in your life.

Carol Brinkman was someone I opened up to. Carol is a hormone specialist and nurse practitioner who has been helping men and women with emotional stability for over 30 years. She helps balance the unbalanced and hot messes like me. At my first appointment, she opened my mind to my low progesterone levels and told me all about what the almighty thyroid gland does. Apparently mine was shot. She became one of my best friends, and she is definitely someone you want to meet. You will find her information in the 'My Favorite Resources' (pp. 114) section of this book.

After seeing Carol and after getting through the holidays that year, I started noticing my waistline was getting smaller. Yes, we were beginning to see the light, people. The combination of hormones and supplements were revealing themselves in my appearance. I was slowly dropping a clothing size, one after the other, after the other. And I wasn't even exercising! My thoughts were becoming clearer, the brain fog had diminished, and the sugar cravings were almost nonexistent. I literally could feel the stress melting away. As the months rolled on, I even began weaning off some of my prescription medications. I went through each one and asked WHY was I taking this? Then worked on them one at a time.

Why was I on a beta blocker for almost 20 years? It wasn't my heart, it was my thyroid. Why was I on an antidepressant for over 15 years? I went to the clinic when my kids were little because I was having trouble sleeping. Hundreds of refills later, I realized all of my kids were grown up and moved out; and I thought, "Why am I still on this?"

As I was healing my body from the inside out, I found an energy I never knew I had.

With losing weight and finding my groove, I started teaching what I learned and I finally developed - confidence. The more I healed and got my life together, the more confident I became to help other women and moms dig out of their holes, just as I had done. Every bit of new education kept me going like hits of dopamine. Every person I helped gave me that much more energy to help the next. Every time I implemented a small change, a positive result always followed.

I finally started to see the light.

BREAKING FREE

Ever since I've learned about functional medicine, my thoughts and beliefs are different - and so is my life. I simply changed my thoughts, which changed my beliefs, and therefore changed my actions. And now I'm experiencing completely different results.

People typically don't just wake up one day feeling depressed with anxiety. Rather, depression can get hold of a person in many different ways. There are so many factors that can become a part of the bigger problem. It's not just one thing.

Here are three that I would like to highlight.

Generational. When a parent suffers from depression, it can be passed to their children through DNA. That's right: A mother's emotional state can actually pass down to her baby at birth. There could also be physical things that happened at birth as well.

Traumatic Events. Depression can also result from an event that was extremely traumatizing. When we don't have tools to handle these events, we resort to tucking them away. Those events eventually plant seeds that fester over time. A lack of confidence and insecurity further weakens a person's ability to deal with the trauma, and emotions start taking over. The cycle continues until a person becomes mentally fatigued. When this fatigue lasts for a period of time, it starts to become "just who you are" and what a person believes to be true about him or herself.

Hormonal Shifts. Depression and anxiety can often be the result of slowly declining hormone levels. This is often due to nutritional depletion, A.K.A. foods and environmental toxins. We will talk more about this in Part 2!

Whether the mental illness is caused by a traumatic event or it's generational, many of the steps towards healing involve making small changes. Along the way, you are bound to think these little changes can't possibly make a difference. But let me tell you, these little things that you think don't matter, do matter. In order for things to change, you have to change. As you go along, you will begin to grasp how important these little things are.

If you feel weak and inadequate, just take smaller steps. You'll soon be surprised at where you find yourself when you keep going.

Are you ready to break free? Please watch The Science of Thought by Dr. Caroline Leaf (link in My Favorite Resources section, pp. 114). Dr. Leaf is an expert regarding the mind-brain connection and how memories affect mental health. This video is a first step to understanding how your past and present thoughts determine your emotional and physical well being.

Being emotionally strong can make all the difference. It has to start with you. Instilling examples of confidence and security in your children involves showing them there is more to life than just working for money and making sure everything looks amazing on the outside. Spend more time together, teach them how to set and achieve goals, praise them right away and set aside time and give them undivided attention. You've got to build them up on the inside. You've got to take the time. I didn't take the time to do this with my Emily.

Sometimes, when people get that label of anxiety and depression, it can become a part of their identity - and those thoughts alone can be heavy. Eventually you believe the diagnosis, then assume the bright orange bottle of pills is going to fix it. But when does it end? Weeks? Months? Years?

Who knew there were studies that show the risk of suicide or suicidal attempts among youths being treated with antidepressants are actually DOUBLE those treated with placebo?[1]

You have to decide when enough is enough.

Who is invested in the results of your choices? YOU ARE. You can choose. I chose to be an advocate for my daughter and myself and the rest of my family. What I was learning empowered me to decide on my own what was right for us, and I became confident in those decisions.

And I never looked back.

If you plan on doing this, I recommend consulting with your provider, as everyone is different. I'm sharing this with you because it was a direction I never knew I could take.

This direction is a choice that you can experience too!

KICKING ITS ASS

We have to learn how to empower ourselves and our children and build them up like it's nobody's business. Ditching those old thought patterns and speaking positive language into their hearts and mind is where it starts. Remember, you are your thoughts, and your subconscious never forgets.

We conscientiously need to be speaking positive and uplifting things into our children everyday. It's not about saying, "Great job" every five minutes, but really stepping into the moment, looking them in the eye and speaking from your heart. Tell them they are beautiful and speak of the good in everything they do.

One of my favorite quotes is,

> "Speak to your children as if they are the wisest, kindest, most beautiful and magical humans on earth, for what they believe is what they will become."
>
> -Brooke Hampton

What if you could teach your children something new that empowers them to process their emotions, so they don't end up buried away to be dealt with later?

In Part 3, I will teach you a mental technique both you and your children can use to shift their thoughts and feelings from ruling their lives. This simple tool can train them to react to their emotions so they don't get stored away and affect them in a negative way. This two-minute technique could change everything.

The countless seminars, webinars and books I've absorbed in

the past eight years have landed us right here. By the time you finish reading this, you will have tools in your tool box you can use to kick anxiety in the ass - a little at a time.

This book is not a one-stop-shop, but a starting point. Every BODY is different and everyone responds differently to different things.

You have to be willing to put in the work and dig deep to the roots.

I wrote this book in an effort to save one busy, stressed out mom who thinks there is no hope. I'm here to hold your hand and tell you that you can do it. It may not be easy, and it may take some time, but it is worth it. My children are worth it. Your children are worth it.

And YOU are worth it.

Are you ready to dive in deep with me and get this party started? Now that you've learned the WHY….let's talk about the HOW.

It's what you've been waiting for.

"Change is painful and uncomfortable, but nothing is as painful as being stuck mentally where you don't belong.

When you start making the little changes is when you can truly start living."

- Stacy Tiegs

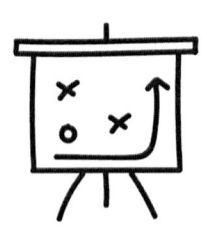

PART 2: THE HOW

Depending on what they are, our habits will either make or break us. We become what we repeatedly do.

- Sean Covey

After starting this journey, some common questions I receive are, "How did Emily overcome her anxiety?" "How did you lose the weight?" Or one of my favorites, "How do you have so much energy?"

Think about it microscopically. Take an ant, for example. If he was building an entire ant hill by himself —we're talkin a two-story Taj Mahal— there ain't no way in hell he could build it overnight. So how does he do it? He does it with tiny, tiny grains of sand over a long period of time. Back and forth, back and forth, focusing on what's right in front of him every-single-day.

I hope you are starting to see the importance of the little things. It's those tiny, tiny decisions you make over a long period of time that will get you to your how.

Let's start by looking at our cells, and we'll see how important these little things are!

THE CRISIS IN OUR CELLS

Our bodies are made up of 50-100 trillion cells. Cells provide structure for the body, take in nutrients from food, and carry out important functions. Cells group together to form tissues, which in turn group together to form organs.[2] Think about your cells being little cars that transport oxygen and nutrients to your entire body. They're kind of a big deal.

They're also constantly being created and destroyed. We have about 300 million cells that die every minute.[3] The rate that our cells die depends on many factors. The more toxins we encounter and the more cells we lose to free radical damage - the worse we feel. When we constantly abuse them with chemicals and that third glass of chardonnay, more cells will die. Many prescription medications affect our cells in a similar way. They can lead to inflammation, which leads to disease. Our goal is to keep our cells as clean and active as possible!

So what's the big deal about toxins? Our bodies don't recognize chemical matter. They don't have a clue how to process them. Think of toxins like little "invaders" that want to take over our bloodstream and mess everything up. Over time, these little invaders can slowly create a place for those uncomfortable side effects. Our bodies are natural and need an intake of natural things in order to create a safe environment. If this buildup of toxins gets to be too much, it can take a serious toll on your liver.

WHAT IF YOUR LIVER WAS THE CULPRIT?

Liver disorders increase the risk of depression and anxiety in young adults. Studies show that teens and young adults with chronic liver conditions suffer from depression and anxiety.[4] Who knew anxiety could have a considerable impact on emotional and physical healing?

The liver is responsible for filtering out all the toxic "junk" we encounter on a daily basis. But just like any other filter, your liver can get backed up. In our cars and homes, we replace air filters every 3-6 months, or they stop working effectively, right? So what's important to know is although drinking water can flush out some toxins, some of them remain in our system and cause a back up, which can lead to numerous side effects.

Think about how you are replacing nutrients that are used or lost. Good health requires that we replace these nutrients to support all our organs, especially the liver. The more chemicals we consume, the greater the toxic load on our body, and the harder our systems have to work.

THE TOXIC OVERLOAD

Today more than ever, our soil, air and water are being stripped of their purity and contaminated by a slew of toxins, and this affects our health more than we know. A lot has changed since great-grandma has been in the kitchen!

SOIL QUALITY: SOUNDS BORING, RIGHT?

Do you know where your food comes from? Do you know how farmers yield their crops? How do they control the weeds around them? Do they hire people to come and pick them by hand or do they save money and spray them with Roundup®?

Glyphosate (AKA-Roundup®) poses major risks to your health. Google it.

The fruits and vegetables grown years ago were loaded with way more vitamins and minerals compared to what we have today. Our soil today is filled with GMO's. A GMO —or genetically modified organism— is a plant, animal, microorganism or other organism whose genetic makeup has been modified in a laboratory using genetic engineering or transgenic technology. This creates combinations of plant, animal, bacterial and viral genes that do not occur in nature through traditional cross-breeding methods.[5]

In a study in The Journal of the American College of Nutrition, researchers report, "Efforts to breed new varieties of crops that provide greater yield, pest resistance and climate adaptability have allowed crops to grow bigger and more rapidly, but their ability to manufacture or uptake nutrients has not kept pace with their rapid growth." [6]

I had to read that twice to really get it. This is what we eat... pest resistance...yummy.

I have friends who actively avoid glyphosate and who have gone all non-GMO, and they experienced a HUGE decline in anxiety.

WHAT'S REALLY IN YOUR WATER?

Our soil isn't the only thing being robbed of nutrients. Most municipal water supplies are processed in such a way that all beneficial minerals are lost. Not only that, but our water is "fortified" with harmful chemicals, like fluorine compounds and trihalomethanes (THMs), arsenic, radium, aluminium, copper, lead, mercury, cadmium, barium, hormones, nitrates, pesticides and heavy metals - just to name a few. Whew! Not only do we make sure to drink eight glasses of this water each day, we use it to cook our food and water our crops for the food we eat.

Maybe it's time to buy that water filtration system you've always wanted. My son-in-law did a test on our tap water in our home, and I almost couldn't believe all the chemicals that showed up in our water! So we added a whole-house water filter, and our water is now clean.

A U.S. Water Drinking Quality Study[7] examined the water supplies of 77 major municipal areas that represent roughly 62% of the U.S. population. The results deem that each area examined was within the EPA's Safe Drinking Water Standards. The real question is, where did these standards come from, and are these limits of chemical and microbial load really optimal? For example, the EPA standard for an acceptable level of trihalomethanes is 80 ppb. Trihalomethane is a class of carcinogenic compounds that includes chloroform.

I think I'll pass on that, thank you very much.

Start questioning these standards as our water quality continues to decline and the contaminants increase.

WHAT ARE YOU BREATHING IN?

Have you taken a breath today? How's the air quality serving you on a day-to-day basis? Most people don't think much about air quality or know how to begin answering that question.

But according to the National Institute of Environmental Health Services, we need to start taking a closer look at the air we breathe and how it affects our health.

Researchers have documented a wide variety of health effects associated with air pollution exposure. These include respiratory diseases (like asthma, allergies, COPD), cardiovascular diseases, adverse pregnancy outcomes (such as preterm birth), and even death.[8]

Everywhere we turn, we are exposed to chemicals that can have a negative affect on our bodies.

ELECTROMAGNETIC FIELDS

These exist wherever there are power lines or outlets, whether or not the electricity is switched on. Magnetic fields are created only when electric currents flow. Together, these make EMFs. Our phones, WiFi, bluetooth, 5G internet, Ipads, television, Alexa, Fit bits, and other devices all emit EMFs. And they all have an impact on our bodies.[9] Also, if you've had x-rays, MRIs, or CT scans, you need to consider the radiation exposure these emit and the negative impact they have on your body.

BLUE LIGHTS

Blue light is a color in the visible light spectrum that can be seen by human eyes. This light is a short wavelength, which means it produces higher amounts of energy. Blue light comes from TVs, smartphones, computers, laptops, tablets, gaming systems, electronic devices, and in LED and fluorescent lighting.[10]

The short wavelengths we get from these electronic devices confuse our bodies and disrupt their natural rhythms.[11] Get some Blue Light Glasses for you and your kids, and limit your screen time as much as possible.

Not only do our devices increase the possibility for cataracts and macular degeneration, they can cause our brains to stop producing melatonin and interfere with our brain and hormone production. This directly affects sleep quality. Plus, lower levels of melatonin contribute to anxiety and depression.[12]

SOCIAL MEDIA

Although social media can offer many benefits, it also has a dark side. Social media can often be the root cause of insecurities, lack of confidence, and other self esteem issues. There are numerous studies that prove social media is frequently a root cause of anxiety.[13]

5G CELLULAR TECHNOLOGY

Cell phone companies began deploying the fifth generation of cellular technology in 2019. Because it is relatively new, there aren't many studies published about its long-term health effects. However, some studies already identify potential risks of exposure to 5G. For example, one review analyzed wireless radiation and states that it not only affects skin and eyes, but will have numerous adverse systemic effects as well.[14] Some people believe 5G is linked to at least 20 ailments, including heart diseases, type-2 diabetes, and mental disturbances, such as depression, anxiety and suicidal tendencies.

THE XBOX

True story - I have a good friend who told me her 11-year-old son would play Fortnight for long periods of time. Fortnite is a survival game where 100 players fight against each other in player-versus-player combat to be the last one standing. It's fast-paced and action-packed.

My friend is a teacher and an incredible mom, but let's get real: It's easy to let our kids play for hours, especially if you don't have neighborhood friends. Well, her son was becoming an absolute nightmare with a negative and angry attitude. She didn't know what to do, so she took his game system away! After a while, he actually thanked her for doing that. He told her, "Mom, I feel better without it."

Gaming also affects our cardiovascular system. The make believe non-realistic adrenalin we get from these affects our health, and over time becomes an addiction. The stress it causes the body will reveal itself in their mood and attitude.

Are you guys still with me?

Good. Now let's jump into skin, shall we?

YOUR SKIN EATS EVERYTHING

Your skin is your body's largest organ, and this organ is like a sponge. Anything you put on it soaks right in and gets absorbed directly into the bloodstream. While our skin does form an excellent barrier to many chemicals, the more we slather on, the more we put ourselves at risk.

Think about those chemicals in sunscreen baking into your skin for hours at a time. Interesting? There was a day when I didn't believe that your skin was absorbent. If water repelled off it then I just assumed everything else did too. Where do you think your lipstick goes after a few hours? Where does the lotion go after you apply it?

Yep. Your skin ate it.

Let's look at a few items you may not have thought of as dangerous or toxic to your health. The question is: Can our bodies tolerate all of this on a daily basis?

- Laundry soap - If you can smell it on your clothes and you're wearing them all day, you are absorbing it.
- Lotions- Can be loaded with parabens, fragrance and other chemicals.
- Soaps- We slather in on daily and even multiple times during the day.
- Makeup - Most are full of chemicals and most women reapply frequently.
- Perfume and body sprays - They weaken our sense of smell and disrupt our endocrine system. Fragrance contains Phthalates that are a known cause of anxiety. There is fragrance in everything these days. Look at your labels.
- Deodorant - Scientists are finding aluminum in breast cancer cells.
- Shampoos/conditioners- Our scalp is porous and absorbs what you're scrubbing in.
- Shavers with instant soap in them- This is a double whammy because you are clearly opening your pores up allowing that fragrant soap to absorb quicker.
- Colored root touch-up sprays- Just like "spray paint"

- Dry shampoo- Powder or spray, if it's sitting on your roots you're eating it.
- Hair dyes- That dye can make its way into your hair fast. Look how long you have to process your hair and the darker colors are worse.
- Nail Polish/acrylic nails- Yes, our nails absorb what is glued to them. Have you heard of formaldehyde or Ethyl Methacrylate? They affect the nervous system and are known to cause cancer and respiratory problems. Look for ones that are better or just go natural and save some money!

Most of these products and things we do on a consistent basis are all a part of our daily routines. Each product may have a small amount of the harmful ingredients that are "regarded as safe", but are they really? How many different products do you use just in the morning? These small, yet harmful, chemicals accumulate and seep into your skin slowly, wreaking havoc on your body. They can disrupt your endocrine function and overload your liver.[15] I call this slow poisoning.

Even products labeled as "natural" or "organic" can have hidden dangerous ingredients. For example, check the label on any of your personal care products and see if it includes the generic term "fragrance". The FDA permits U.S. manufacturers to legally hide hundreds of synthetic chemicals in this one word without revealing what those ingredients are. These can include petrochemicals and phthalates. Phthalates are industrial chemicals used to soften PVC plastic and as solvents in cosmetics and other consumer products. They can damage the liver, kidneys, lungs, and reproductive system.[16,17] Yes, I used to be a perfume/Glade® candle smell freak too. That was until I realized what spraying fragrances directly on my neck was doing to my thyroid. This led to many side effects, and I'm so grateful I ditched all that and found Thyromin™.

Most personal care products are a concoction of chemicals. In very small doses, the FDA claims these chemicals as GRAS (generally recognized as safe). However, the FDA does not take into consideration the quantity of chemicals we load on our bodies throughout the day.

The average woman applies 300 chemicals before she goes to work. That does not even include the preservatives and chemicals we consume in our breakfast, lunch or dinner. If you added all of it up in the course of one day, you'd get an idea of why you have side effects. Not only that, but common sense says that no amount of carcinogenic, endocrine disruptors is a safe amount for me and my family. I'll pass on those too.

When was the last time you read the ingredient list on your favorite fragrant body wash, make up or lotion? Start your own research today, and you'll be appalled at the chemicals your body is sucking up on a daily basis through your skin.

I highly recommend the Environmental Working Group website to check the toxic level of products you use. They also have a phone app that is really handy for scanning products before you buy! Check the 'My Favorite Resources' section for links (pp. 114).

CHEMICALS TO AVOID

Below is a list of some of the most common chemicals to be on the lookout for. I challenge you to dig a little deeper for yourself on all of these. Trust me, I didn't believe it either.

- Fragrance
- Phthalates
- Sodium lauryl sulfate (SLS) and sodium laureth sulfate
- Parabens
- Diethanolamine (DEA) and triethanolamine (TEA)
- Triclosan
- Bisphenol A (BPA)
- Toxic metals: lead, nickel, mercury, cadmium
- Nanoparticles
- Talc
- Benzene
- Preservatives
- Carrageenan
- Propylene glycol (PEG)
- Aluminum

- Titanium dioxide
- Fluoride
- Toluene
- Artificial color
- Formaldehyde
- Oxybenzone
- Mineral oils
- BHA and BHT
- Coal tar dyes: p-phenylenediamine and colours listed as "CI" followed by a five digit number
- DEA-related ingredients
- Dibutyl phthalate
- Hydroquinone
- Petroleum
- Natural or Organic Labels - Get the scoop: www.fda.gov/Cosmetics/ResourcesForYou/Industry/ucm388736.htm#7

COULD A DEFICIENCY BE THE PROBLEM?

When we think about our bodies and what they need to survive, we tend to think about basic things: food, water, clothing, shelter, (and wine of course). But many of us forget about other things our bodies need to survive.

Our bodies are made up of elements; primarily oxygen, carbon, hydrogen, nitrogen, calcium, and phosphorus. About 0.85% of our bodies are composed of potassium, sulfur, sodium, chlorine, and magnesium. These elements are essential for survival.

So what happens when we don't get enough of these elements to replace what is lost or deficient? These deficiencies appear in your body as symptoms. Maybe you feel tired all the time, or you're more stressed than you should be. Do you often get headaches for no apparent reason? Often, you don't feel sick, but you just feel "off" in some way. For many people, these small symptoms are so normal, they don't even notice them. In truth, "normal" should mean feeling energetic, positive, clear-headed, and motivated. Anything outside of this can be classified as a symptom.

THE GUT-BRAIN CONNECTION

Believe it or not, most of what goes on in your brain is heavily influenced by the health of your gut. It took years for me to understand this connection. This is because many of the hormones and neurotransmitters that affect your mental state, such as serotonin and dopamine, are actually produced in the gut. Many studies about the gut-brain connection demonstrate the importance of a healthy intestinal microflora.[18]

> In fact, more than 90% of the body's serotonin, "the happy hormone", is produced in the gut. Serotonin contributes to positive mood and feelings of well-being and happiness. Maintaining good gut health can actually help reduce depression, stress, anxiety, and serotonin-related health problems.[19][20] It is so important we take care of our gut, and this begins with diet.

Diet affects our blood, organs and the vital microbiome in our gut. Because 75% of our immune system resides in our gut, this directly affects our quality of life, especially as we age. So many of us just think about getting through the day with eating to get full and not even thinking about where the real nutrition is. We should really be focusing on how we want to feel 5-10 years from now. The good news is, it's never too late.

We are almost to the best part. Is your head spinning yet?

THE GUT & YOUR HORMONES

Hormones control just about everything in our bodies. They play a role in our emotional state, regulate what keeps us calm when we are stressed, and affect our energy levels. An imbalance in the endocrine system can cause hormonal shifts that also result in anxiety, mood swings, depression and emotional roller coasters. Remember the chemicals we talked about earlier? These disrupt normal endocrine function and literally rob our bodies of these critical elements.

Progesterone is another key hormone that plays a significant role in mental health and how we handle stress. Just a slight drop in progesterone due to hormonal imbalance can affect mood and well-being.[21]

Did you know women with low progesterone levels and men

with low testosterone are prone to anxiety? Estrogen helps to stimulate the production and transportation of serotonin around the body, and prevents its breakdown. Therefore, when estrogen levels and serotonin levels are low, an unstable mood and anxiety can develop.

When Emily got married and was trying to conceive, she saw Carol Brinkman, my BFF hormone specialist. Her blood work revealed that her progesterone levels were completely depleted. Even with that news, it was such a relief to finally understand the root cause! I'm grateful she went in, as this assisted in making a grandchild for me.

Let's not forget about thyroid problems. Your thyroid gland is located on your neck and controls your metabolism and plays a role in regulating other hormones. Did you know an underactive and overactive thyroid gland can trigger bodily symptoms that are similar to panic attacks? Think about where you spray perfume. Chemical fragrances are endocrine disruptors. If you use perfume, you are giving your thyroid gland a direct daily blast of chemicals that can cause dysfunction in adults and children.

Like other glands in the body, the thyroid doesn't function by itself; it works with other endocrine organs, like the adrenals, pituitary, pancreas, liver and reproductive organs. When these other organs are overworked or overstimulated by stress, food allergies, poor diet and/or lack of sleep, it causes the thyroid to work even harder to compensate, which can contribute to stress and anxiety. This is why it's so important to monitor your hormones and get them checked if you suspect something is off.

What if it were that simple? Go in for a simple diagnostic blood panel with a specialist to get the answers you need. Sadly, the hormone ranges that most doctors consider "normal" are far less than ideal. There are critical things many practitioners do not even test for.

Take the time to see a specialist. Ask around for a referral or do your research to find a doctor who understands all of this. If you can't find a doctor, check the 'My Favorite Resources' section (pp. 114) for a suggestion.

> ## A NOTE ABOUT THE PILL
>
> Both progesterone and estrogen are known to affect mood, and the hormonal birth control pill contains synthetic versions of these hormones. This study has found that women with a history of depression are at increased risk of experiencing mood swings and anxiety when taking hormonal birth control.[22]

LEAKY GUT SYNDROME

Leaky gut syndrome is a digestive condition that affects the lining of the intestines. In leaky gut, gaps in the intestinal walls allow bacteria and other toxins to pass into the bloodstream. Unfortunately, many doctors and healthcare professionals do not recognize leaky gut syndrome (LGS) as a diagnosable condition.[23]

It is important to note that when we consistently eat foods that cause inflammation in our gut, leaky gut syndrome results. This leads to seepage of toxins, microbes, antibodies, and undigested food particles from the intestines into the bloodstream. The result of this includes a lot of physical issues, but you may be surprised to learn it also affects your emotional well-being.

PARASITES: EVER THOUGHT YOU COULD HAVE THESE?

The definition of a parasite is "an organism that lives in or on an organism of another species (its host) and benefits by deriving nutrients at the other's expense". If your child is hyperactive, has dark circles under her eyes, grinds or clenches his teeth, constantly picks his nose, wets the bed, has restless nights, cries for no reason, pulls her hair out, or has recurring headaches, I would consider looking into parasites as the cause.

Humans get parasites from our water, food, pets, raw fish, undercooked meats, and other things. Some parasites create no harm, but some can lead to severe illnesses. Some parasites can even mess with your central nervous system and cause a wide variety of side effects. Get your poop tested, people! The Ova and Parasite test is the best and most accurate. They actually take a sample of your stool and look at it under a microscope for living parasites and their eggs. Can you imagine? It may require more than one test to see if you have them. They are sneaky. See the 'My Favorite Resources' section (pp. 114) for the best book on this.

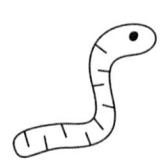

WE REALLY ARE WHAT WE EAT

Most people know our physical health is directly affected by what we eat. But did you know that what we eat also determines our emotional health too? If this is a new concept for you, I suggest you read through this next section carefully. I will discuss the major food-related contributors to mental health issues, but it's important to note that this is not a comprehensive list.

FOODS THAT CONTRIBUTE TO ANXIETY & DEPRESSION

CAFFEINE

Caffeine stimulates dopamine release in the brain. This pleasure hormone is the reason many people crave a caffeine boost and also contributes to its addictive nature. Ever wonder why a good chocolate bar can ease depression? Yep, that's the dopamine coursing through your veins.

It's important to keep in mind that caffeine only brings temporary relief. Although caffeine can immediately improve mood with a dopamine high, this causes a depletion of serotonin production over time, which will ultimately make you feel worse. Decreased serotonin production can lead to depression as well as other issues, such as decreased immune function.[24]

Studies show that caffeine also causes an increased release of cortisol, the stress hormone related to the fight-or-flight response in the body. In a nutshell, this means caffeine contributes to stress reactions. This stimulant effect may include feelings of nervousness, nausea, light-headedness, jitteriness and yes, even anxiety.[25]

Did you know caffeine can cause nutrient depletion of important nutrients, like vitamin B6, and interfere with nutrient absorption of essential minerals, including calcium, iron, magnesium, and B vitamins? This also affects physical and emotional health.[26]

If you're suffering through anxiety, you may want to reconsider your morning cup of coffee, tea, or soda. Try herbal tea, water, or kombucha instead.

Check out the beverages with the highest amount of caffeine:

- Death Wish® coffee - 651 mg
- Starbucks® 20 oz. venti coffee - 415 mg
- Dunkin Donuts® 20 oz. coffee with turbo shot - 395 mg
- Spike® 16 oz. energy drink - 359 mg
- Mr. Hyde® 16 oz. Power Potion - 350 mg
- Wired® X344 16 oz. energy drink - 344 mg
- Redline Xtreme® 8 oz. energy drink - 316 mg
- Bang® 16 oz. energy drink - 300mg
- Spike® Shooter 8.4 oz - 300 mg
- Cocaine® 8.4 oz. energy drink - 280 mg
- Biggby® Red Eye 16 oz. brewed coffee with espresso - 274 mg
- Peet's® 16 oz. brewed coffee - 267 mg
- Panera® 16 oz. frozen mocha - 267mg
- Redline Princess® 8 oz. - 250 mg
- Redline® 8 oz. energy drink - 250 mg
- Shock® Coffee 8 oz. Triple Latte - 231 mg
- Starbucks® 16 oz. grande caffe Americano - 225 mg

There are many more, but just one of these quick pick-me-ups can trigger anxiety and all the other negative effects of caffeine.

REFINED SUGAR

Here we go! The detrimental effects of sugar are hard to ignore because sugar is hidden in everything! The addictive nature of sugar can cause an increased state of anxiety similar to that seen during withdrawal from addictive drugs. Long-term consumption of sugar can cause more widespread anxiety and impair the body's ability to effectively cope with stress.[27]

> Fact: sugar has been known to be as addictive as cocaine. As an addictive drug, when we don't have it for a period of time, we experience actual withdrawal symptoms. Sugar crash symptoms include mood swings, heart palpitations, difficulty concentrating, and fatigue.[28]

Two-hundred years ago, the average American ate only two pounds of sugar a year. In 1970, that figure jumped to 123 pounds of sugar per year. Today, the average American consumes almost 152 pounds of sugar in one year. This is equal to 3 pounds (or 6 cups) of sugar each week![29] The recommended maximum serving is around 6 teaspoons a day.

In the brain, excess sugar impairs both cognitive skills and self-control. Because of its drug-like effects in the reward center of the brain, having a little sugar often stimulates a craving for more.

Increased sugar in the blood can increase insulin resistance in the body. Extreme levels of sugar can interfere with neurotransmitters in the brain responsible for stabilizing moods. This often leads to depression, anxiety, hyperactivity, and more mood-related issues. Hearing that alone should make you toss the Pop Tarts® and Froot Loops®. They do make great fire starters.

Because overconsumption of sugar triggers imbalances in certain brain chemicals, it creates a vicious cycle. The more a person consumes sugar to numb emotions, the worse those symptoms of sadness, fatigue, and hopelessness become. I mean, I used to have a fridge full of every variety of pop and juice known to man. It's no wonder we were all a mess.

You also have to beware of hidden sugars. Of course we know the obvious sources, such as cakes, cookies, biscuits, and other sweets. But sugar is also hidden in foods that may seem healthy at first glance, like fruit juices, smoothies, dried fruit, crackers, breads, etc. Most cereals are FULL of hidden sugars.

Our bodies turn 100% of the carbohydrates we eat into glucose. This affects blood sugar levels as quickly as an hour or two after eating. So if you find yourself (or your child) on an emotional swing, take a look at what you ate an hour or two ago. Foods that turn into sugar include simple carbohydrates, like bread, rice, pasta, potatoes, starchy vegetables, fruit, yogurt, and milk.

> Think About It: Does your toddler throw temper tantrums? Did you just give them a cup of juice, a sucker, chocolate milk or a piece of bread two hours ago? Could their behavioral symptoms actually be a sugar crash?

Learn to read labels. Sugar may be disguised with various different names:
- Fructose: found in fruits, juices, and honey
- Galactose: found in milk and dairy products

- Glucose: found in honey, fruits and vegetables
- Lactose: found in milk, made from glucose and galactose
- Maltose: found in barley
- Sucralose: made up of glucose and fructose and found in plants

FRUIT JUICES

Although fruit juice may seem like a healthier option, it is loaded with sugar just like soda and other store-bought beverages. Fruits and vegetables owe their sweet taste to natural fructose. Fructose stimulates neural pathways that affect how the brain responds to stress, which can have detrimental behavioral effects, including the worsening of symptoms related to depression and anxiety.[30]

Does this mean fruit is bad for you? Not necessarily. When we drink fruit juice the fiber has been removed. Fiber protects us from absorbing too much fructose, so when we remove the fiber, we put our bodies at risk of overconsumption. Fiber makes you feel full and we need 30 grams per day.

Go ahead and eat the apple (with the peel) instead of drinking apple juice. If you really want an occasional cup of fruit juice, it's best to make it at home and drink it fresh. If you love juicing, limit the amount of fruit you put into your green juices. Stick to the 80/20 rule (80% vegetables/20% fruits) and you'll be good to go. Fiber is everything!

ARTIFICIAL SWEETENERS

If you think you're doing better by passing on the real sugar and using artificial sweetener instead, you may want to rethink that choice. I used to think those little pink and blue sugar packets were good for you. Sugar substitutes may help you cut calories, but you really need to be careful!

Aspartame is the most common artificial sweetener found in foods and low calorie beverages. Like sugar, it interferes with the normal production of serotonin in our brains.[31] Studies of healthy adults who ingested reasonable daily amounts of aspartame had more irritable mood and exhibited more symptoms of depression.[32] Aspartame is also believed to be responsible for headaches, insomnia, and anxiety, and has been linked to certain forms of cancer.

Fortunately, there are some safer choices when you need a bit of sweetener in your coffee or tea that we will cover in Part 3.

GLUTEN

Gluten is a protein found in wheat, barley and rye products. Gluten sensitivity is very common. However, gluten does not only affect those with documented gluten allergies or sensitivities. Studies show that gluten affects the nervous system even in people without Celiac disease or gluten sensitivity. These symptoms include depression, anxiety, and other mood disorders.[33] Try omitting gluten for 1-2 weeks and watch what happens.

A scientific review involving over 1,000 study subjects found that there was a direct relationship between depression and gluten consumption. Gluten causes inflammation in the gut and can upset the natural microflora that helps govern our emotional state. Researchers say that gluten elimination may represent an effective treatment strategy for mood disorders and recommend further research into gluten elimination as part of a protocol for depressed individuals.[34] What if this one little thing alone you could change the way you feel?

If you suffer from depression or another mood disorder, you may want to consider trying a gluten elimination diet for a period of time. The good news is that most patients report a relief from symptoms within just a few days of cutting gluten from their diets. Could it really be that simple? Maybe. Remember, sometimes those little changes we make can add up to big changes.

> Elimination Diet:
>
> Phase 1 - Elimination: Stop eating foods you suspect trigger your symptoms for a short period of time, typically 2–3 weeks. This may include gluten, dairy, caffeine, nuts, corn, and soy.
>
> Phase 2 - Reintroduction: During this phase, slowly bring eliminated foods back into your diet. Introduce each food group individually over a period of about 2–3 days, and closely monitor for symptoms.

PROCESSED FOODS

These "foods" are easy and cheap, rarely expire, and should be avoided as much as possible. Some common processed foods include cereals, cheese, milk, bread, cookies, crackers, granola bars, dried fruit, popcorn, lunch meats, jerky, baking mixes, convenience foods (such as soups, noodles, freezer dinners, lunch packs, etc.) This list could go on and on, but hopefully you get the picture. Generally, processed foods are high in sugar, gluten, fat, and sodium, as well as a bunch of other additives and preservatives.

With the lack of any nutrients, and all those chemicals in processed foods, it's no surprise that they are harmful to the natural bacteria and microbes in the gut.[35] The most highly processed foods contain loads of preservatives to give foods a longer shelf life. Sadly, many of these preservatives are directly linked to an increase in anxiety and depression symptoms.[36]

So next time you're at a family BBQ, avoid grilled hot dogs and opt for a salad and other fresh foods. Fresh, natural, whole foods made from scratch are the best. If a food doesn't mold within five days on your counter, then you should be skeptical of preservatives and other chemicals that may be present.

Preservatives and Food Additives to Avoid:
- Monosodium Glutamate (MSG)
- Artificial food coloring
- Sodium nitrate
- Trans fat
- Artificial flavoring
- Yeast extract
- High fructose corn syrup
- Sodium benzoate - For example, one study found that combining sodium benzoate with artificial food coloring increased hyperactivity in three-year-old children.[37] Another study showed that consuming beverages containing sodium benzoate was associated with more symptoms of ADHD in 475 college students.[38]

ALCOHOL

We all enjoy an occasional drink, right? But what happens when that one glass of wine at dinner turns into three glasses of wine and dessert?

Some people resort to consuming alcohol as a means of dealing with anxiety issues. Because alcohol is a depressant, it has a relaxing, sedative effect, and people often use it to unwind. However, using alcohol to treat anxiety is a strategy that backfires. According to the Substance Abuse and Mental Health Services Administration (SAMHSA), anxiety is a mental health disorder that can actually be caused by prolonged drinking.[39] Studies show that excessive drinking can lead to the rewiring of the brain and make an individual more prone to anxiety.[40]

Alcohol also has various effects on the nervous system. The toxic effect of alcohol on nerve cells can result in hypersensitivity, increased heart rate, lowered blood sugar levels and acute dehydration.[41]

If you struggle with anxiety or depression, you may want to skip that nightcap or casual drink out with friends. While it may offer you temporary relief from your anxiety, you will likely worsen your symptoms in the long run.

DAIRY

Remember those "Got Milk" ads that popped up during commercial breaks on TV shows in the 90s? The marketing strategy was very strategic. They used our favorite cartoons, athletes, and superstars that would be reminding us consistently to drink up. But is milk really a healthy drink?

About 10% of adults are lactose intolerant, and even more have difficulty digesting the casein found in cow's milk. Oftentimes allergies and sinus issues go away when omitting dairy. Let's not leave out its impact on children. Young girls are getting their menstrual cycles earlier and developing breasts faster from all the hormones they ingest in regular milk and meat. If you add up all the processed foods we eat and all the hormone disruptors in our food and personal care products, the results and consequences are definitely not good.

The truth is, dairy can wreak havoc on the digestive system. I don't know about you, but bloating, diarrhea and constipation don't sound fun to me.

SODA

Most people already know that soda is not good for you. The sugar and caffeine high from soda makes our brains crave more and more. What's absolutely crazy is that statistics show that the average American drinks 44 gallons of soda each year, and children between the ages of 12-19 drink the most. We know that soda affects our bodies and can contribute to obesity, diabetes, tooth decay, dehydration, heart disease, kidney problems, and more.[42] But many people are not aware of the effects of soda on mental health. This is a big deal.

We've already covered the dangerous effects of sugar on our bodies, so we need to take a look at how much sugar is contained in our favorite soft drinks. The U.S. Department of Agriculture (USDA) recommends limiting sugar to less than 10% of your daily caloric intake. But the American Heart Association disagrees, recommending half that amount. For the average American, this equates to about 6-12 teaspoons a day. Sodas and canned energy drinks contain the equivalent of about 9-30 teaspoons of sugar per 12 oz. can!

Knowing this, the answer is not to reach for that diet soda either. The dreaded aspartame is the most common sweetener in diet soda.

Soft drink consumption also contributes to obesity, tooth decay, cardiovascular disease, diabetes, osteoporosis, hypertension, and more. You already know it, so I won't dwell on it any more - soda is just bad for you. It affects every single body system and negatively impacts the health of your brain and your mood.

If you struggle with anxiety—or any other health issue for that matter—I strongly suggest you eliminate soda from your diet. When my husband's knee pain went away when he quit drinking pop and replaced it with water, it was quite the eye opener.

FRIED FOODS

We all know fatty, fried foods are bad for us. This is not news, right? But did you know they also contribute to depression?

Most fried foods are cooked in partially hydrogenated oil. Anything cooked in hydrogenated oil can potentially contribute to depression. You see, proper brain development and maintenance requires essential fatty acids (EFAs). Omega-3 fatty acids, such as fish oils, are vital for brain health. Unfortunately, trans and saturated fats crowd out EFAs in the brain. This increases the risk of developing Alzheimer's disease, dementia, and mental illnesses, including depression.[43][44]

Saturated fats, found in meat products and dairy, can also clog arteries and prevent blood flow to the brain. This not only contributes to poor brain health, but can also increase the risk of high blood pressure and heart disease.

Building a healthy brain begins before birth. Eating a lot of trans fats during pregnancy can affect your baby's brain development. Isn't it amazing that we can actually start taking care of our children's mental health before they are even born?

Moderation is key. The next time you find yourself at your favorite burger joint, opt for the kiddie size fries instead of the super-size. Or buy grilled chicken instead of fried. There are so many little things you can begin to think about!

FOODS HIGH IN SODIUM

Remember the fat-free craze years ago? The reality of this fad was that most foods that are fat free are actually higher in sugar and/or sodium. The overconsumption of sodium can lead to obesity, high blood pressure and water retention.

Facts are facts, and too much sodium in the diet can have a negative impact on the neurological system. A low-salt diet may improve anxiety, irritability, depression, fatigue, insomnia, and migraine headaches.[45] One study showed that participants who consumed salty foods prior to going to bed took longer to fall asleep, experienced more sleep disturbances, and had lower quality of sleep (fewer hours of REM sleep), dissatisfaction with sleep, and more fatigue and drowsiness the following day.[46]

A reasonable amount of salt is essential for maintaining good health. Salt provides essential electrolytes that help maintain fluid balance and facilitate the transmission of nerve impulses. Sodium also helps your body regulate blood pressure and absorb chloride, amino acids, glucose and water. But too much salt in your diet can send you down a slippery slope of anxiety, panic and depression. So just go easy on the salt shaker.

FOOD DYES

These are a huge culprit when it comes to behavioral issues. All those colorful chips and candy are making us bounce off the walls. Product manufacturers use additives like food dyes to enhance flavor, appearance, texture, and shelf life of various foods. But people are finally catching on to the dangers of food dyes. Austria and Norway have banned the use of artificial food dyes, and European health authorities require a warning label on foods that contain dyes. Meanwhile, the FDA in the U.S. has yet to open their eyeballs to this.

So just how dangerous are artificial food dyes? The three most widely used culprits, Yellow 5, Yellow 6 and Red 40, contain benzene, a known carcinogen.[47] Research also shows a direct association between food dyes and attention deficit problems in children and adults, including hyperactivity, learning impairment, irritability, and aggression. These symptoms were noted both in populations with a diagnosis of Attention Deficit Hyperactivity Disorder (ADHD) as well as healthy individuals with no mental diagnosis.[48]

Adults with ADHD show a direct relationship to depression and anxiety. The dysfunctional problems and social avoidance that results from disorders like ADHD frequently cause depressive symptoms and increased stress levels.[49] This is profound. When I hear of more and more people cutting dyes out of their diet these days, it gives me hope. More people are starting to read labels and do their own research.

I had the pleasure of helping a friend's 12-year-old daughter with some emotional things she was going through. Right away, I asked her what her diet was like and she told me all of her favorite foods were red! Red gummy bears, red fruit snacks, and red drinks. After working with them for several months and taking out these food dyes, her mood changed significantly.

IT ALL STARTS IN THE MORNING

Have you ever noticed that when you eat junk for breakfast, you have a tendency to eat more junk during the day? If you set your day up with a wholesome, healthy breakfast, you will be more likely to carry on that trend throughout the day.

It is especially important for children to eat breakfast. A nutritious breakfast will benefit their cognitive function and performance at school.

As you read this, keep in mind that the recommended maximum sugar intake for children ages 2-18 years old is 25 or fewer grams per day. Below are some typical breakfast choices children are faced with on a daily basis:

- 2 plain Eggo® waffles with 1/4 cup real maple syrup = 51 grams
- 2 Frosted Cherry Pop Tarts® = 34 grams
- 1 Cinnabon® cinnamon roll = 58 grams
- 1-cup serving of Frosted Flakes® cereal = 13.8 grams
- 1-cup serving of Cap'n Crunch® cereal = 16 grams
- 1 Strawberry Nutri Grain® cereal bar = 12 grams
- 1 Quaker® Oats instant oatmeal packet = 12 grams
- Peanut butter & jelly on white bread = 17-25 grams

I hope your jaw is dropping here. Mine was when I learned the reality of what we were eating. I mean, we felt lucky to be eating Lucky Charms® and we knew there must be fruit in Froot Loops®, right? And who wouldn't feel like a captain eating Cap'n Crunch®? Wow. lesson learned.

If you want to motivate your children to eat less sugar for breakfast, you should model the behavior yourself. Let your children see you eating the same breakfast as you serve them (or at least use the same ingredients). In time, your child will be less excited about sugary foods and more in favor of the healthier options.

SCHOOL LUNCHES

School lunches are the easiest answer for some families, but unfortunately, the average school lunch leaves much to be desired when it comes to providing proper nutrition for your children. The illustration below depicts a typical lunch served in our schools today.

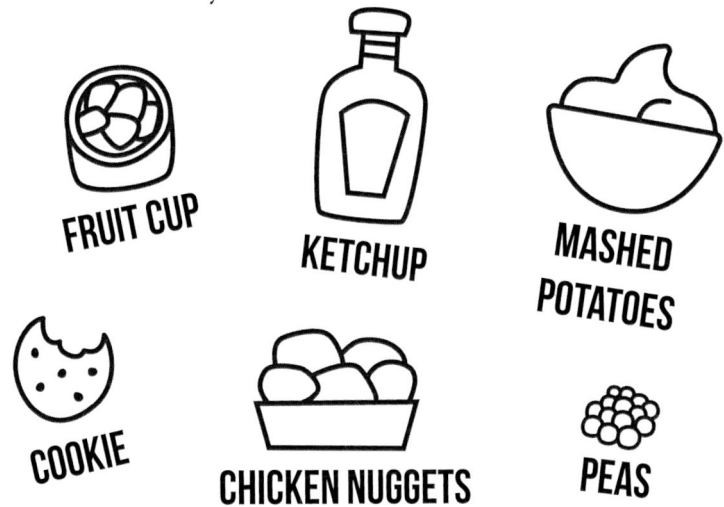

FRUIT CUP

KETCHUP

MASHED POTATOES

COOKIE

CHICKEN NUGGETS

PEAS

Let's break each item down with its sugar content.

- Chicken Nuggets: Not much sugar
- Cookie: 12 grams of sugar
- Fruit cup: 12-15 grams of sugar
- Ketchup: 8 grams of sugar in ¼ cup
- Peas: 8 grams of sugar in 1 cup

Total Sugar Content: 40 Grams, and this doesn't include a juice or milk box. That's a lot of sugar and it only constitutes one meal of your child's day. EEK!

Aside from the sugar, let's have a look at the other ingredients that could be lurking in that lunch:

- Potato Flakes: Sodium bisulfite, BHA and citric acid, contains 2% or less of each of the following: Monoglycerides, partially hydrogenated cottonseed oil, natural flavor, sodium acid pyrophosphate, butteroil
- Chicken nuggets: Typically made with mechanically separated chicken using the bits and parts of chicken carcasses that are not sellable. Those nuggets may contain only 50% meat and the rest is fat, ground bone, blood vessels and connective tissues. Yuck!
- Canned Peas: While peas are low in saturated fat, cholesterol and sodium and are a good source of protein, thiamin, folate, iron, dietary fiber, vitamin A, vitamin C, vitamin K and manganese, most of this nutrition is lost in the canning process. The peas that were once healthy and vitamin-packed provide little to no actual nutrition.

FAST FOOD

Experts estimate that approximately 12-15% of a child's daily calories comes from fast food. No wonder childhood obesity is becoming a norm among American youth. According to the CDC National Center for Health Statistics Prevalence of Obesity Report of 2015-2016, obesity prevalence was 13.9% among 2- to 5-year-olds, 18.4% among 6- to 11-year-olds, and 20.6% among 12- to 19-year-olds.[50]

Just take a look at the nutrition facts of the average McDonald's® Happy Meal:

- 450 - 710 calories
- 13 - 27 grams of fat

- 52 - 98 grams of carbohydrates
- 18 - 58 grams of sugar
- 10 - 26 grams of protein

Moms, we have to do better here. Convenience food is messing with your child's health and neurological development. Not only do these choices affect their performance at school, they also contribute to your child's attitude and mental health as well.

WHERE IS THE REAL NUTRITION?!

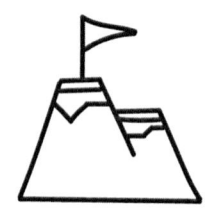

PART 3: WHERE DO I START?

If the previous section has your head spinning, don't worry. It was so overwhelming for me at times too. We are now going to focus on the good, better, and best of specific food choices.

Fortunately, many of the physical and emotional issues caused by foods will improve or subside within a short period of removing the "culprit" foods from your diet.

Before you venture out on your next shopping trip, here are a few tips:

- Don't bring your kids shopping with you. It's very challenging to read ingredients on labels and nurse your two children at the same time.
- Depending on where you live, there are many healthier stores to go to. Whole Foods®, Trader Joes®, Aldi®, Coborns® and even Target® have healthier and organic options.
- Send your husband; he will always stick to the list.

- Buy fresh, organic food as much as possible.
- Always plan ahead weekly and bring a list of items you need.
- Avoid aisles in the store that have a lot of temptations for you.
- Order online if you can and pick up. Amazon has Fresh Delivery or shop their Pantry Delivery.
- Never shop hungry. Slam some water and get full. If I happen to be hungry while grocery shopping, I will always open a bag of something I plan to buy, like almonds, and eat while shopping. I'm kind of a rule breaker.
- Have your EWG phone app downloaded and ready to go. This will help you make healthier choices. Here's how: Click to watch.

> ### ORGANIC, NON-GMO? WHICH IS BETTER?
>
> Non-GMO essentially means none of the ingredients in a product have been genetically modified. But that doesn't necessarily mean it's good. It doesn't tell you where the food came from or how it was grown/produced. Certified organic, by definition, also means a food is non-GMO. Plus, it means that the food contains no pesticides, herbicides, antibiotics, and other nasty "additives". So yes, look for food that is non-GMO, but the ultimate peace of mind comes when the label says it's certified organic.

FOOD CHOICES TO CONSIDER

You will love this next section that includes a few of my favorite things. Of course, cooking everything from scratch using whole foods is your best option. But let's be real...most of us will do that only on occasion and most of the time will reach for something more convenient. In this section, I tried to include a bit of both. Is every option absolutely perfect? No. Are they better? Yes. Your kids WILL get used to the change. We have to start somewhere!

Now that we've discussed what not to eat, let's look at foods that you should be eating.

OATMEAL

GOOD

Oats Overnight

Worthy Superfood Blendie Bowls

BETTER

Quick Cooking Steel Cut Oats

Qiá Superfood

BEST

Make Ahead Instant Oatmeal Cups

Yield: 8 servings

Prep Time: about 5 minutes for 8 breakfasts!

Ingredients

5 cups old-fashioned rolled oats

1/2 cup packed light brown sugar

1 tsp. ground cinnamon

1/2 tsp. kosher salt

Optional add-ins:

Unsweetened dried fruit (bananas, raisins, apples, cherries, strawberries)

Coconut flakes

Chopped nuts (pecans, almonds, walnuts, etc.)

Seeds (chia or flax seeds)

Instructions

Combine oats, sugar, cinnamon, and salt in a large bowl and stir to combine.

Pour ½ cup servings into sandwich bags and add desired toppings to each.

When ready to serve, pour contents of one baggie into a bowl and add 1/2 cup of boiling water. Stir to combine, and let sit for 5 minutes before eating.

CEREAL

I get it. Some kids (and even adults) just love cereal. While most cereals are processed and loaded with sugar, there are some good-for-you options available. Do your homework and read those labels. Here are a few favorites:

GOOD

Nature's Path EnviroKids Cheetah Chomps

Nature's Path Sunrise Crunchy Maple

BETTER

Nature's Path Fruit Juice Corn Flakes

Purely Elizabeth

Keto Nut Granola

BEST

Gary's True Grit Einkorn Flakes Cereal

Three Wishes Grain Free Cereal

MILK

Cow's milk is meant for cows. But I know many children—and even adults—love their milk, especially with a bowl of cereal. You can wean off of cow's milk to a healthier plant-based milk by adding just a bit of the plant milk to the cow's milk. Gradually increase the amount you add, and your kids will barely notice when you make the switch.

When looking for milk alternatives, the fewer ingredients the better. Avoid carrageenan and as many "gums" as you can, especially if you currently have digestive issues. Gums are thickening agents, but they can have undesirable side effects.

A WORD ABOUT GUMS IN FOODS

Guar gum is a fiber that comes from a plant. Xanthan gum is produced by fermenting a carbohydrate with Xanthomonas campestris bacteria, then processing it. Both of these gums can have effects on digestion, which may or may not be desirable. Gum arabic comes from the sap of the acacia tree. This gum may actually support the growth of beneficial gut bacteria. None of these are particularly bad for you, but in excess, guar gum and xanthan gum may cause bloating, diarrhea, or constipation.

PLANT-BASED MILK ALTERNATIVES

So Delicious Organic Unsweetened Coconut Milk

Pacific Foods Organic Unsweetened Coconut Milk
Good Karma Plant-Powered Flax Milk

COFFEE & TEA

While small doses of caffeine are acceptable, caffeine addiction can wreak havoc on your body and brain. (See the section about caffeine on pp. 114 for more information.) If you are caffeine-dependent, I strongly suggest you work to decrease your daily intake. Better yet, stop using caffeine for a few weeks and take note of how you feel after your body completely withdrawals. Chances are, you'll experience an increase in energy and may decide to never go back.

Green tea contains the amino acid theanine, which may have anti-anxiety and calming effects by increasing the production of serotonin and dopamine.[51] Choose green tea for your caffeine fix or as a healthy replacement for soft drinks, coffee, or alcoholic beverages.

Chamomile tea has been popular for centuries as an herbal remedy because of its anti-inflammatory, antibacterial, antioxidant, and relaxant properties. A recent study found that chamomile is effective at reducing anxiety symptoms with no side effects.[52]

For those who love a warm cup of coffee or tea in the morning, here are a few favorite options:

GOOD

Bulletproof Organic Coffee
Peak Performance Organic Decaf Coffee

BETTER

Rishi Organic Loose Leaf Earl Grey Tea

Rishi Organic Peppermint/Sage Tea Bags

Slique Ocotea Oolong Cacao Tea

BEST

Rishi Organic Jasmine Green Tea Bags

Numi Organic Jasmine Green Tea

Organic India Tulsi Green Tea

Traditional Medicinals Organic Chamomile Tea

STARBUCKS®

The sugar content in just one of Starbucks' most popular drinks is well over the maximum daily recommended allowance for sugar, not to mention the combined caffeine hit.

STARBUCKS® RUN SUGAR FACTS:

Aside from the calories and fat contained in these drinks, it's really the sugar that's the culprit. This dose of sugar starts your day with an insulin spike. Many people consume these drinks on a daily basis. Could this be why you feel so short-tempered and stressed-out?

16 OZ. GRANDE BEVERAGE	CALORIES	GRAMS OF SUGAR
Beast Mode Frappuccino	430	59
Caffè Vanilla Frappuccino	430	69
Caramel Frappuccino	410	64
Caramel Macchiato	240	32
Chai Créme Frappuccino	360	50
Chai Tea Latte	260	42

CREAMER

Some of us can't go without the cream or flavoring in our coffee or tea. Fortunately, there are a few healthy options to replace the chemical and sugar-laden brands.

GOOD

Nut Pods flavored liquid creamers - contain gums

BETTER

Karma Kafe Keto Creamer (contains butter and is higher in calories)

BEST

Terra Soul Coconut Milk Powder

Laird Superfood Coconut Milk Creamer

PANCAKE & WAFFLE & MUFFIN MIXES

Skip the processed frozen options and pancake mixes that are loaded with sugar. Even if you don't make pancakes from scratch, there are so many better options available.

GOOD

Bob's Red Mill Gluten-Free Pancake Mix

Keto & Co Pancake Mix

BETTER

Simple Mills Pancake Mix

Birch Benders Paleo Pancake & Waffle Mix

Keto Muffin Mix

Simple Mills Muffins Variety

BEST
Einkorn Pancake & Waffle Mix
Gluten-Free Einkorn Pancake Mix

SYRUP

Even though natural syrups are still high in sugar, it's better to avoid corn syrup and any additional additives.

GOOD
Ningxia Berry Syrup

BETTER
Organic, Non-GMO Maple Syrup

BEST
Healthier Flapjacks and Waffles:

Spread a teaspoon of good quality organic coconut oil on each pancake or waffle and top with a sprinkle of Monk Fruit Powdered Sugar. You can also combine 1 tablespoon of pure maple syrup with plain non-fat Greek yogurt and use as a dip. You'll use much less syrup and it tastes delicious!

EGGS

One egg has only 75 calories, but contains 7 grams of high-quality protein, 5 grams of fat, and 1.6 grams of saturated fat, along with iron, vitamins, minerals, and carotenoids. The egg is a powerhouse of disease-fighting nutrients, like vitamin D, lutein and zeaxanthin.

Eggs also contain tryptophan, which is an amino acid essential to the creation of our happiness hormone, serotonin.[53]

Eat them scrambled, over easy or even boiled and peeled for a grab-and-go snack.

> QUICK AND MEAL IDEA:
> Choose a coconut or cauliflower-based wrap (see the Breads section) and add scrambled eggs, a sprinkle of cheese, and a dash of salsa or ketchup. Roll up and hand to the kids on their way out the door!

FRESH FRUIT

Fruit is an inexpensive, simple option. A pile of fruit contains a lot of natural sugar.

GOOD

<u>Bananas</u>

Lower blood pressure
Anti-Inflammatory
Fight depression and anxiety
Reduce risk of stroke
Heart-healthy
Ease constipation
Help prevent kidney cancer
May help curb sugar cravings

BETTER

<u>Apples</u>

Support healthy body weight
Heart-healthy
Decrease risk of diabetes
Promote healthy gut bacteria
Support a healthy brain
Detoxifying to the liver

BEST (THESE FRUITS CONTAIN LESS NATURAL SUGAR)

<u>Melons (watermelon, honeydew, cantaloupe)</u>

Heart-healthy
Support kidney health
Boost energy
Support healthy weight management
Good for skin
High in antioxidants

<u>Berries (strawberries, blueberries, raspberries, etc.)</u>

High in antioxidants
Heart-healthy
Improve blood sugar
Lower blood pressure
Cancer preventive
Help with weight management
Anti-inflammatory
May lower cholesterol

<u>Wolfberries</u>

Protect the eyes
Provide immune system support
Protect against cancer
Promote healthy skin
Stabilize blood sugar
Decrease depression and anxiety
Improve sleep
Prevent liver damage

YOGURT

Many yogurts contain healthy probiotics that improve gut health, but we need to watch for sugar content and unwanted additives. Pro tip: Buy plain, unsweetened yogurts and add in your own honey and fruit for sweetness.

GOOD
- So-Delicious Coconut Milk Yogurt
- Chobani Less Sugar Greek Yogurt

BETTER
- Siggi's Strained Non-Fat Yogurt
- Dannon Oikos Non-Fat Greek Yogurt

BEST
- Stonyfield Organic Yogurt
- Fage Total 0% Greek Yogurt

BREAD/WRAPS

Some of us are addicted to bread, rolls, tortillas, and other floury items, but remember, refined flour turns into sugar within minutes after you eat it.

GOOD
- Dave's Killer Bread

BETTER
- Bfree Gluten Free Pita Bread

BEST
- Nuco Duo Organic Coconut Wraps
- Plant Power Sandwich Thins
- Cauliflower Flatbreads

CONDIMENTS

Condiments are a great way to add flavor and variety to your foods, but they can also pack on the calories. I trust anything from Primal Kitchen. Their sauces and dressings are fabulous and contain no hidden sugars or additives.

> Ingredient Lesson: Although Heinz® sugar free ketchup contains no added sugar, it is sweetened with the artificial sweetener, sucralose. This controversial sweetener is made from sugar in a multistep chemical process in which three hydrogen-oxygen groups are replaced with chlorine atoms. Beware: This substance may damage good gut bacteria. Don't be fooled; buy a better option.

GOOD

Heinz 75% Less Sugar Ketchup

BETTER

Coconut Aminos (Coconut aminos are a great alternative to soy sauce, but be careful if you are watching sodium intake.)

Bragg's Coconut Aminos

BEST

Primal Kitchen BBQ & Steak Sauce

Primal Kitchen Organic Unsweetened Ketchup

Muir Glen Organic Salsa

COOKING OILS

We need oil to help cook and season our food, right? Fortunately, fats are not bad for you as long as you choose the right kinds. Avoid margarine and processed oils in favor of better options with the kinds of fats our bodies need. Avoid corn, canola, peanut, soybean, safflower, sunflower and shortening oils as well.

GOOD

<u>Vital Farms Pasture-Raised Butter</u>

<u>Epic Organic Pork Lard</u> (pork fat)

BETTER

<u>Ancestral Supplements Grass-Fed Beef Tallow</u> (beef fat)

<u>Botanical Beauty Organic Palm Oil</u>

<u>La Tourangelle Avocado Oil</u>

BEST

<u>Nutiva Organic Unrefined Virgin Coconut Oil</u>

<u>La Tourangelle Organic Extra-Virgin Olive Oil</u>

SUGAR ALTERNATIVES

Below are some alternatives to sugar. These are handy for baked goods, coffee or tea, or pretty much anything to which you'd normally add sugar. Some alternative sweeteners take a bit of getting used to, but once you stop eating sugar and make the switch, your taste buds will adjust faster than you expect.

Stevia is a natural sweetener from a plant and is likely the healthiest option. Xylitol and erythritol are sugar alcohols and are a little harder to digest, but tend to have a taste more similar to table sugar. Other options, like maple syrup, molasses and honey, are slightly better than regular sugar, but should still be used sparingly. As with most things, moderation is key.

GOOD

Truvia Brown Sugar

Whole Earth Baking Sugar

BETTER

Organic Coconut Sugar

BEST

Organic Stevia Powder

Stevia Liquid Sweet Drops (your kids will love these)

Monk Fruit Extract

PASTA

Fortunately, most grocers carry several varieties of gluten-free pasta. You can find pasta made from almost any grain, like rice, corn, or quinoa. Some pastas are made from beans, lentils, and chickpeas for an added boost of protein and other vitamins.

GOOD

Explore Cuisine Organic Pasta

BETTER

Banza Chickpea Pasta Variety Pack

Einkorn Spaghetti Pasta

BEST

Organic Black Bean Spaghetti

Chickapea Organic Chickpea/Lentil Spaghetti

SPAGHETTI SAUCE

Most spaghetti sauces contain loads of sugar, so it's vital to read the label. These are a few that my family enjoy. Or do some canning and make your own!

GOOD

365 Everyday Value Spaghetti Sauce

BETTER

Rao's Homemade Marinara Sauce

BEST

Muir Glenn Spaghetti Sauce

FLOUR

Flour is naturally a yellowish color, so it is bleached using chemicals like chlorine and benzoyl peroxide. The process destroys most of the nutrients, so it is then "enriched" with synthetic vitamins that our bodies can't absorb.

GOOD

High Fiber Coconut Flour

BETTER

Organic Almond Flour

BEST

Einkorn Flour

Einkorn: A Seed to Seal Story

Difference between einkorn and regular wheat: Einkorn has gluten, but it may be a healthier version, making it easier to digest compared to the gluten found in modern wheat. Einkorn is a diploid like most plants, meaning it has two sets of chromosomes, while modern bread bread has six sets.

PEANUT BUTTER

Choosy moms shouldn't choose sugar-laden processed peanut butter.. Many famous brands are loaded with sugar as well as other unnecessary ingredients. When it comes to nut butters, stay away from hydrogenated palm oil or soy. Impure peanut butter costs less and has a longer shelf life, but you get what you pay for. The only ingredient needed to make REAL nut butter is nuts and maybe a little salt. Also consider almond butter. It has more vitamins, minerals and fiber than peanut butter.

GOOD
Peanut Butter & Co. Old Fashioned Peanut Butter

PB Fit Organic Peanut Butter Powder

BETTER
Justin's Classic Almond Butter

Santa Cruz Organic Dark Roasted Peanut Butter

BEST
Better Almond Butter

Barney Almond Butter

ON-THE-GO

Sometimes we just want a quick grab-and-go snack to take on the run. Check out some of my family's favorites.

SNACK BARS

GOOD
Bearded Brothers Organic Food Bars

That's It Blueberry & Apple Fruit Bars

BETTER
Nuts & Berry Antioxidant Snack

Kate's Real Food Granola Bars

BEST
Chocolate Coated Wolfberry Crisp bars

Einkorn Granola

FRUIT SQUEEZE PACKS

GOOD
Noka Superfood Pouches Variety Pack

BETTER
Mamma Chia Strawberry & Banana Squeeze

BEST

Squeeze Station Make your own squeeze packet with this inexpensive machine. Then you know exactly what you are getting.

CHIPS

Look for chips with fewer ingredients and always consider the oil they are fried in as well.

OILS TO AVOID:
Canola, Soybean, Sunflower, Corn, Safflower, Grapeseed, Margarine.

OILS TO CHOOSE:
Butter, Tallow, Lard, Coconut Oil, Extra-Virgin Olive Oil, Avocado Oil, Palm Oil

GOOD
- Beanfields Variety Pack
- Boulder Avocado Potato Chips
- Malt Vinegar Boulder Canyon
- Off the Eaten Path (my favorite)
- Garden of Eaten Sesame Blues Corn Tortilla Chips

BETTER
- Pop Chips
- Barnana Plantain Chips

BEST
- Cauliflower Pretzels
- Cauliflower Crackers

MEAT SNACK STICKS

- Vermont Uncured Turkey Pepperoni Sticks
- Primal Turkey Stick
- Epic Beef Sticks

NUTS & SEEDS

Nuts and seeds make great snacks. Not only are they convenient, but a small handful can provide a good source of protein, fiber, and unsaturated fats. They also contain vitamins and minerals, like omega-3 fatty acids and vitamin E. The fiber and protein in nuts will help you feel fuller longer, and keep you from munching on lower-quality calories later. Nuts are calorie-dense, so just remember portion control.

Pumpkin Seeds are a great source of potassium, which may help reduce stress and anxiety. They also provide zinc, which is essential for brain and nerve development and may help improve mood.

Almonds contain a lot of fiber as well as vitamin B and E. Studies show that the antioxidant activity of vitamin E is key for reducing anxiety and stress.[54]

Walnuts also contain high levels of vitamin E, along with alpha linolenic acid and phenolic compounds, which help prevent mental decline and even assist in reducing mild depression. They also contain melatonin, which helps regulate natural sleep patterns.

Cashews provide a valuable source of the depression-fighting hormone tryptophan, as well as magnesium, which supports mood.

Brazil Nuts are high in selenium. In fact, 1 ounce of Brazil nuts supplies more than the recommended daily allowance of selenium. Studies show this element may improve mood and reduce symptoms of depression. It is also a vital nutrient for proper thyroid function.

Pecans contain dietary fiber, which helps your body cleanse itself of toxins. They also contain essential vitamins, minerals, and antioxidants.

OTHER SNACK OPTIONS

YumEarth Organic Fruit Snacks

Bare Medleys Dried Fruit

Dried Wolfberries

Food to Live Raw Organic Almonds

Hu Kitchen Dark Chocolate Bars Variety Pack

SOFT DRINKS & ENERGY DRINKS

I am so grateful there are healthier options to name-brand sodas and energy drinks!

GOOD
Zevia Zero Calorie Energy Drink

BETTER
Zevia Zero Calorie Soda

Zevia Organic Tea

BEST
NingXia Nitro Energy Shots

NingXia Red Metabolism-Boosting Superfood Drink

Zyng Health Energy Drink

BOTTLED WATER

Did you know that a little dehydration can cause moodiness and make you tired? Lack of water affects every system in your body, and without it your systems start to malfunction. It affects your hormones, the way you use your brain and blood flow.[55] Water is absolutely vital for just about everything your body needs to run right. We should aim to drink half your bodyweight in ounces per day.

Bottled water is convenient, but many brands are no better than chlorine-treated tap water. Plus, all the extra plastic waste is terrible for the environment. Save money and purchase a countertop water filter and some good quality refillable water bottles. If you have to buy bottled water, look for the brands below.

GOOD
Nestle Pure Life

BETTER
Fiji

Evian

Essentia Ionized Water

BEST
Berkey Water Filter

Make water taste better with these Vitality Electrolytes. Electrolytes are chemicals that conduct electricity when mixed with water. They regulate nerve and muscle function, hydrate the body, balance blood acidity and pressure, and help rebuild damaged tissue.

PROTEIN

Protein helps stimulate the production of dopamine (the feel-good feeling) to help combat anxiety. Every cell in the human body contains protein. You need protein in your diet to help your body repair and make new cells. Protein is also important for growth and development in children, teens, and pregnant women. Protein powders are a great way to supplement protein into your diet. Just be careful and find a good quality protein, and stay away from fillers.

The following should never be in your protein powder: Casein + WPC, gluten, dextrins/maltodextrin, artificial sweeteners, skim milk powders/milk solids, soy protein, vegetable oils and fats, added fibers.

WHEY Isolate protein is 90% protein. It's jam packed with amino acids, including the two biggies, tryptophan and glutamine. Your body does not produce these, but they are vital.

Tryptophan: Plays a role in the production of serotonin.

Glutamine: Is a precursor to GABA, which regulates neurons that keep you calm in your central nervous system.

RECOMMENDED DIETARY ALLOWANCE FOR PROTEIN:

AGE/GENDER	GRAMS OF SUGAR
Children ages 1-3	13
Children ages 4-8	19
Children ages 9-13	34
Girls ages 14-18	46
Boys ages 14-18	52
Women ages 19-70+	46
Men ages 19-70+	56

GOOD

Orgain Organic Plant-Based Protein Powder

BETTER

Pure Protein Complete Chocolate

Pure Protein Complete Vanilla Spice

BEST

Garden of Life Organic Whey Grass-Fed Protein Powder

Ass Kicking Anxiety Shake: Combine 1 banana, 1 scoop of whey protein, ½ cup water or almond milk, ½ cup greek yogurt, and ½ cup ice and blend till smooth. Yum!

DARK CHOCOLATE

Many women will rejoice to learn that chocolate does, in fact, help reduce stress and anxiety. I'm so glad there is a real study on this one. It shows that chocolate helps reduce stress by lowering stress hormones cortisol and epinephrine and decreasing the body's response to the brain signals of stress.[56][57]

When looking for the perfect chocolate, the darker the better. Look for chocolate that is 70% or more cacao. Dark chocolate also contains sugar and fat, so satisfy that craving with a small serving of 1 to 3 grams.

BEST OPTIONS

Choc Zero

That's It

Taza- Wicked Dark

Hu Vegan Chocolate Bars

Hu Single Bar

With anything on these lists, if you can't always buy the best, buy the good; and then work your way to better a little at a time.

NUTRITIONAL SUPPLEMENTATION

Most of us are mineral deficient. Vitamins and minerals are considered essential nutrients, especially if you have anxiety. They are the driving force in the body and our energy supply. They help heal up bones, heal wounds, and bolster our immune system. They also convert food into energy, and repair cellular damage.

MINERALS

CALCIUM

Calcium is the most abundant mineral in the body. In addition to supplying our teeth and bones with what they need, calcium plays a role in cardiovascular health and maintaining communication between the brain and other parts of the body. A calcium deficiency in the diet can result in the body stealing this vital mineral from our bones, causing osteoporosis.[58]

Eat:

- Leafy green vegetables, like broccoli, kale, cabbage and okra
- Organic soybeans and tofu
- Nuts and seeds, especially almonds and sesame and chia seeds
- Sardines and salmon
- Yogurt

MAGNESIUM

Magnesium is a natural muscle relaxer, which helps immensely with anxiety. It's a nervous system relaxant and mineral that assists with fear, irritability, and restlessness. We hold on to so much tension within our muscles, and this is a super-healthy and easy way to create calmness.

It improves brain function and supports those neurotransmitters that send messages to your brain.[59] It also helps regulate healthy blood pressure and supports the immune system. It is great for building strong bones and heart and maintaining normal blood sugar.

Eat:

- Dark chocolate
- Avocados
- Nuts, like almonds, cashews, and peanuts
- Legumes, such as kidney and black beans
- Organic soy milk, tofu, and edamame beans
- Whole grains, such as oats, barley, buckwheat, brown rice, and quinoa
- Bananas
- Spinach

POTASSIUM

Potassium functions to regulate fluid balance and control the electrical activity of muscles in the body, including the heart. It supports healthy blood pressure, cardiovascular health, and strengthens bones and muscles.

Eat:

- Fruits: bananas, oranges, cantaloupe, honeydew, apricots, grapefruit, prunes, tomatoes, raisins and dates
- Sweet potatoes

- Mushrooms
- Beans, such as white, lima, pinto, and kidney beans
- Peas and lentils
- Cucumbers, zucchini, eggplant, and pumpkins

SODIUM AND CHLORIDE

Sodium and Chloride provide vital electrolytes that maintain fluid balance in the blood. Salt gets a bad rap, but we actually need a healthy amount of salt in our diets to ensure proper blood volume, maintain healthy blood pressure, and regulate the pH of body fluids.

Eat:

- Seaweed
- Rye bread
- Vegetables like tomatoes, lettuce, celery, beets, and carrots
- Olives
- Fresh sauerkraut (not the canned stuff)
- Wild-caught salmon (not farm-raised)
- Certain dairy products, like ricotta cheese, plain yogurt, and eggs

PHOSPHORUS

Phosphorus is necessary for building bones and teeth, as well as building proteins that function to grow and repair cells and tissues in the body. It plays an important role in the processing of carbohydrates. Phosphorus is essential to the healthy function of the nervous system, kidneys, heart, and muscles.

Eat:

- Chicken, turkey, pork, and organ meats
- Seafood
- Dairy products, such as cottage cheese and yogurt
- Seeds, such as sunflower and pumpkin seeds
- Nuts
- Whole grains, such as oats, barley, buckwheat, brown rice, amaranth, and quinoa

SULFUR

Sulfur is found in nearly all human proteins, such as collagen and keratin, which supply the building blocks of tissues and organs. These proteins strengthen bones and teeth, as well as skin, hair, and nails. Signs of sulfur deficiency include sagging skin, thin, fragile nails, and painful joints.

Eat:

- High-protein foods, like beef, poultry, fish, and eggs
- Nuts, including peanuts, Brazil nuts, almonds, peanuts, and walnuts
- Seeds, such as pumpkin and sesame seeds
- Peaches, apricots, and figs
- Beans, like black, white, and kidney beans
- Vegetables, such as asparagus, broccoli, Brussels sprouts, red cabbage, leeks, onions, radishes, and turnips
- Certain whole grains: pearl barley, oats, wheat, and flour made from these grains
- Beer, cider, and wine

PROBIOTICS

Studies show there is a direct communication between your gut and brain. (See the section on The Gut Brain Connection, pp. 114) Taking care of the microbiome in your gut with foods and probiotics can help with anxiety. Probiotics help balance the friendly bacteria in your digestive system. They prevent and treat bowel problems, improve mental health conditions. Certain strains also contribute to heart health and reduce the severity of certain allergies and eczema.[60] All my kids and grandchildren take probiotics.

VITAMINS & SUPPLEMENTS

VITAMIN B12

What if a simple vitamin is all you needed? Vitamin B12 benefits mood, energy levels, the cardiovascular system, hormone balance, and digestion. It is a vitamin my family will never be without. Deficiency in vitamin B12 can cause a variety of psychiatric symptoms, from anxiety and panic to depression, chronic fatigue, and even hallucinations.

Our bodies do not store water-soluble B vitamins, and most people don't get enough of them through diet, so it is important to take them daily as a supplement. It is also important to make sure you purchase a good source of vitamin B12 because most cheap drugstore vitamins are not absorbed by the body.

VITAMIN C

Vitamin C is a strong antioxidant that combats oxidative stress in the body. This may help reduce the risk of many health issues, including heart disease, hypertension, and high cholesterol. Vitamin C also improves the absorption of iron, which is normally poorly absorbed by the body. Vitamin C supports the immune system by improving white blood cell function and production.

Low vitamin C levels have been linked to an increased risk of mental disorders, such as dementia; while a high intake of vitamin C has been shown to provide a protective effect. Low levels also contribute to schizophrenia, anxiety & depression.[61]

VITAMIN D

Vitamin D, also known as the sunshine vitamin, is 100% necessary for your body to absorb calcium and helps regulate blood pressure and blood sugar. Vitamin D also helps regulate neurotransmitters in the brain, such as dopamine and serotonin, thus having a direct effect on mood. Vitamin D deficiency, especially in geographical areas with periods of reduced sunlight, can result in seasonal affective disorder (SAD), depression, anxiety, and other mental illnesses.[62] My kids get vitamin D in their stockings for Christmas. That's how important they are.

Are you always on the go? An incredible multivitamin for those looking for a one-stop-shop that is loaded with all the essentials is Master Formula - all-in-one with 4 capsules.

L-THEANINE

L-Theanine is an amino acid that can be found in Green Tea. When taken with supplements, this study showed that it can have an incredible impact for those with anxiety.[63]

These KidScents Unwind packets contain L-theanine as well as magnesium and are a must have for anxious moms and kids.

TURMERIC

The benefits of turmeric are too good not to include, and the studies are profound. Turmeric is a spice commonly used in Indian and Southeast Asian cooking. The active ingredient in turmeric is curcumin, which may help lower anxiety by reducing inflammation and oxidative stress. A 2015 study found that curcumin reduced anxiety in obese adults.[64]

Turmeric is easy to add to meals. It has minimal flavor, so it's easy to sneak into soups, smoothies, curries, and casserole dishes. It comes in real vegetable form, pills or liquid.

> If you are feeling overwhelmed, it's okay. I completely understand. There are so many things you can do, so to make it easy, simply start with ONE thing.

WHAT WILL BE YOUR ONE THING TO START?

> Brain trick: When you feel that anxious trigger coming... count backwards in your head 5,4,3,2,1 and find an anchor thought. Find a thought that makes you really happy and practice this. This will trick your brain and you won't focus on the problem anymore but rather getting done what you need to get done.

MANAGING - ACTION ITEMS

So now that we know about foods, supplements, and how they can affect our bodies, here are other things to consider. Again, anxiety comes in all forms and there are many ways to manage it. Along with food strategies, there are mental strategies we can utilize too.

Here is my favorite mental strength technique that helps me daily with little things that hold me back. It's something you can practice daily so you can be the master of your brain.

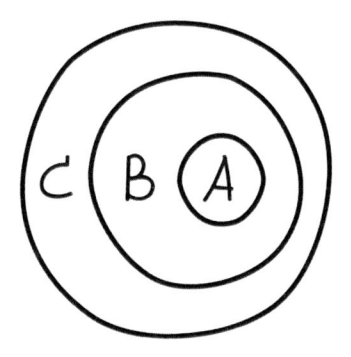

A-CIRCLE MENTAL STRENGTH TECHNIQUE

Developed by Stacey Herman

I want you to visualize three circles, small, medium and large. Like a red target practice sign and label them A, B and C. The small circle is your A, medium circle is your B, and the large circle is your C-circle. Everything that's in your A-circle is mentally what's running your show. Your A-circle is who makes decisions for you and who's in charge. There is no right or wrong answer. It can be a person, thought or emotion.

Inside the B-circle are people, emotions or thoughts that influence you, but don't make decisions for you. The C-circle is everything else that doesn't matter. Keep one thing in mind, the only person in charge of your circles, is YOU. You own them and you get to dictate how you let things in mentally.

Can you remember a time when something was running the show for you in your A-circle and prevented you from doing something you wanted to do? Let's use anxiety as an example. Let's say you were diagnosed with anxiety and depression. Your subconscious tells you that you can't do something because of your anxiety and all the side effects attached to that. Now, visualize moving that anxiety mentally into the B-circle. It's still there, but when you move it into your B-circle, you no longer have to allow it to make decisions for you, kind of like setting it on a shelf for a while so you can finish what you were set out to do.

The point is, don't allow it to rent space in your head (A-circle), because YOU want to make all the decisions, not anxiety. The C-circle is for all the drama, negative thoughts and all the other messy thoughts that really don't matter. That thought or friend you thought was a friend really isn't and now you can choose where she fits in your life.

This is an especially great exercise for children who endure any kind of bullying. Was there ever a time when your child was bullied and you had no idea how to help him or her? This tool can help them see that they don't have to accept the hurtful words of others and allow them to affect their decisions and behaviors. They can take the thoughts or words of others and deliberately put them into their C-circle because they don't matter—ever.

This is so empowering because whoever is doing this technique gets to choose what they are allowing their A-circle. They get to choose what becomes important and everything that's not.

AROMATHERAPY

Your sense of smell is your only sense that has a direct connection to your brain. Essential oils from plants provided our first line of defense thousands of years ago. If they are distilled the right way, they become therapeutic. They are referred to in the Bible hundreds of times, so that's pretty solid. They are so simple to use and can support all of our body systems, including emotions. Studies show that using essential oils can have a calming effect on nerves and can be effective for treating a variety of anxiety disorders.[65]

You need to know there is a difference among essential oils, and they are not all created equal. You see them almost everywhere you go. But as with most things, you get what you pay for!

THERE ARE FOUR GRADES OF ESSENTIAL OILS:

- Grade A: Therapeutic, grown from the best plants and steam distilled in the optimum way to ensure the therapeutic value of the oil stays perfect with all of the plant's powerful constituents. Contain no additives or fillers and have no expiration date.

- Grade B: Food grade. May contain chemicals, carrier oils, solvents, pesticides, or fertilizers. Many are labeled "Do not ingest" or "Do not take internally".

- Grade C: Perfume/fragrance oils. Likely contain solvents and up to 95% alcohol. These are what you find in commercial bath products, candles, and air fresheners.

- Grade D: Floral water, which is the leftover water from steam distillation of plants. It may smell nice, but it has no therapeutic value and may contain harmful residues.

This will make you shake your head. Are you ready? Companies are allowed to label essential oils as '100% Pure Therapeutic Grade' if they contain as little as just 6% of essential oil. It just goes to show you that you can't always trust the labels.

Do your research. Understand that if you buy a drugstore essential oil for a few bucks, you are probably just getting a useless liquid with a nice aroma. But that liquid could contain other chemicals and contaminants that do not belong on your body or in your lungs.

My choice is Young Living. Their oils are 100% therapeutic grade and have a Seed to Seal® promise. This assures you that the essential oils contain absolutely no contaminants, chemicals or additives. Young Living is over 25 years old and I wholeheartedly value the integrity of Gary and Mary Young that paved the way for all of us for years to come.

Almost all essential oils support emotions in some way. To use them, simply inhale from the bottle, place in a diffuser, or wear topically on your wrists, the back of your neck or on the bottoms of your feet.

Here are just a few that I recommend for emotions.

- Lavender
- Valor® - Emily's Favorite
- Rose
- Ylang Ylang
- Bergamot - Emily's Favorite
- Lemon
- Orange

- German Chamomile
- Melissa
- Jasmine
- Clary Sage
- Neroli
- Basil

AROMA FREEDOM TECHNIQUE

One of my favorite quick relaxation techniques is AFT The Aroma Freedom Technique Video. Created by Dr. Benjamin Perkus, it is a proven method to initiate a positive outlook and attitude. AFT taps into our sense of smell and gently shifts our awareness away from negative thoughts, feelings and memories. Once we can shift in a new direction, we can move forward and create the life we truly want. The Aroma Freedom Technique book is an incredible resource to help you learn to do the technique anytime you want. (See the Resources section, pp. 114 for a link to purchase.)

RAINDROP TECHNIQUE

I highly recommend experiencing the Raindrop Technique. This technique was invented by Gary Young in the 1980's. It's designed to bring balance to the body with its relaxing and mild application. It involves the application of essential oils to your back and feet without hard pressure or trying to force the body to change. The process is very relaxing and helps to release emotions of all kinds. If you have had serious trauma, regular Raindrop Technique treatments could help you overcome the emotional setbacks.

To find a Certified Raindrop Technique Specialist, go to Raindrop Education - CARE program for more information.

CBD

CBD, or cannabidiol, is a natural substance that comes from the hemp plant. It supports your vital endocannabinoid system, which regulates many functions in the body to keep everything running the way it should.

This system plays a part in the regulation of:
- Appetite
- Digestion
- Sleep
- Pain perception
- Memory
- Reproduction/fertility
- MOOD
- Energy regulation
- Inflammation
- Pleasure/reward

You can purchase CBD just about everywhere now (even in gas stations!) Trust me, it's not just a trend that should ever leave. This plant was growing everywhere until 1937, when the government ruled that it should be "illegal" because it comes from the Cannabis plant, the same genus from which marijuana is obtained. People back then were paying up to $1,000 for a small amount of this natural remedy because it worked so well.

However, we now know that CBD and the THC found in marijuana are not the same, and they have different effects on the body. Unlike THC, CBD does not produce the "euphoric" sensation and will not get you stoned. But it does act on the endocannabinoid system in different ways.

As with all natural products, not all CBD is created equally. Some sources contain traces of THC that can show up in drug tests. You need to know from where the plants are sourced and if they are organic and free of pesticides. If you are looking for CBD that is pure and 100% free of THC - [Nature's Ultra is where to start.](#)

To make it simple: Our bodies have cellular receptor sites that want what is in the cannabis plant. There is much to learn and study on this plant, but for now, just know that CBD is safe and can be an incredible tool for regulating mood.[66] See resources for Dr. Oliver Wenker's CBD Book.

CRAFTING

One of my favorite craft activities is making bracelets. They are simple and fun for everyone and can definitely help reduce anxiety. There is something very calming about touching the beads, which have healing properties of their own. Add a little essential oil to the lava beads, wear around your wrist, and the oil will absorb into your skin and keep you relaxed.

Check out the 'My Favorite Resources' section for a link to purchase the kits I use to make diffuser bracelets.

EXERCISE

Did you know that exercise relieves anxiety and depression with just a 10 minute walk? This is just as good as a 45-minute workout. The studies show that exercise can work really quickly to elevate depressed moods in many people. Yes, it's temporary, but that quick walk or a simple activity can offer hours of relief, just like taking an aspirin for a headache.

There is evidence that physically active people have less anxiety than those who are less active. Exercise helps the brain cope better with stress. People who get regular vigorous exercise are 25% less likely to develop depression or anxiety disorders over the next five years.[67]

HOBBIES

Creating positive memories with your kids is priceless. Finding a hobby can help those who suffer from anxiety, depression or chronic pain. It eases stress and can increase happiness and protect the brain.[68] Even a simple activity, such as coloring in a book, can be therapeutic. Sign up for a dance class, take a horse riding lesson or learn how to play an instrument.

LAUGHING

There's nothing like a good laugh. Science has proven laughing on a regular basis has numerous positive psychological effects. Force yourself to laugh. Watch YouTube videos or movies that make you laugh. Just smiling can improve your mood but laughter can release stress. It increases oxytocin and dopamine levels that make us happy.

LIGHT THERAPY

If rainy days get you down, or if long winters leave you feeling blue, a portable White Light can help. Studies show that a little white light can eliminate or reduce the amount of antidepressant medication needed to alleviate anxiety or depression.[69] Light therapy may offer a great alternative for people who want to avoid antidepressants altogether. Simply turn it on and sit near it, or bring it to the office and use it at your desk.

MEDITATION

I had no idea breathing was such a big deal. What if you tried this simple free tool from Pamela Hunter?

A PERSONAL EXPERIENCE STORY FROM PAMELA HUNTER ABOUT MEDITATION:

"Meditation was a foreign word to me while anxiety was very familiar, as I referred to myself as the "happy depressed person". I began practicing yoga to help my anxiety in 1999 and eventually learned that meditation was part of the 8 limbs of yoga. It was through my breathing practices that meditation became real to me. My anxiety was coming from outside influences all around me, and my breath was deeply rooted inside of me. When I learned how to breathe —mindfully breathe— I could feel myself returning to a peaceful truth inside myself. I would sit, breathe, and meditate. My definition of mindful meditation is awareness of our breath, our physical sensations in our body, our emotions, our mind, and our environment. Meditation is the stillness of our mind while being at ease in our body. Eventually, through the practice of yoga, breathing, and meditation, I could recognize with awareness when my thoughts would begin to get hold of me and anxiety would begin to surface. Then I would practice breathing, which led me into meditation."

Mindful breathing is a wonderful way to begin your meditation practice. Simply notice your breath. Do you feel your breath moving in and out of your nose? Simply notice. Is your breath long or short? Deep or shallow? Smooth or uneven? Simply notice without judgment. Can you feel your breath in your belly? Is your belly moving while you breathe? As you breathe in, your belly rises. As you breathe out, your belly falls. Notice the rhythm of your breath. Feel your feet on the earth as you breathe. Take out your Peace & Calming® essential oil. Breath in peace and breathe out calm. Breathe. Practice. Meditate.

Get the <u>Simply Being</u> Phone App for a guided relaxation meditation session you can do daily (see Resources section).

PRAYER

Praying can be profound and highly recommended. Find a Bible or a Daily Devotional Book that resonates with you. Tune into words from Dr. Carolyn Leaf who has studied the brain for over 30 years, "It has been found that 12 minutes of daily focused prayer over an eight-week period can change the brain to such an extent that it can be measured on a brain scan. It's comforting to know that God can do all things if you just ask.

READING

When you read, it brings you to a different place and it can take your mind off of everything else. It causes your brain to focus on something different.

YOGA

Yoga is an incredible way to calm the mind. I used to think it was only for the "hippie" people out there, and I wanted no part of it. That was until I went to a yoga retreat with some friends and met Ed Daily. Spending three days on a mat quieting the mind didn't seem very "fun" at the time. Let's just say, at the end of those three days, my mind was calm and others noticed. I highly recommend it. It wasn't as I expected it to be.

Studies about the emotional health benefits of yoga are numerous. The calming breathing and stretching involved can help alleviate stress, anxiety, and depression.[70]

"Yoga has been known for hundreds of years for its physical and psychological, emotional and spiritual benefits. In recent years, these ancient sciences have been more well-studied for the benefits on the body and mind. Learning the methodology to help reduce anxiety is relatively easy and effective if practiced consistently over time."

-Ed Dailey

"Yoga. It's so much more than being on a mat. When yoga found me 15 years ago, it changed my life. I took a community ed class, and I was about to discover that this first class would lead me on a journey of self-healing and discovery, and soon would save my life...Shortly after I went to my first class, I went through the darkest point in my life and found that yoga opened up a gateway of grace, forgiveness, and healing.

"At first, I thought I had to be flexible to attend a yoga class. I quickly realized that's like thinking I had to be good at guitar before I took guitar lessons. My yoga teacher once told me, 'Where you are is exactly where you should be.' This little message created a flood of grace for myself (and others) that I have carried forward in my life.

"Yoga is different for many. Some are drawn to a fitness-gym-type of yoga, where it is more fast-paced. Others are drawn to a quieter atmosphere where there are less people, and possibly slower paced. Some prefer to do yoga in the privacy of their home by themselves, or with an online teacher. Whatever type of yoga resonates with you is where you belong."

"When entertaining a practice of yoga, remember this: Shop around for a yoga teacher/mentor who resonates with you. Remember, not all teachers and studios will be a good fit for you, and that's okay. Keep looking until you find what resonates with you. You will know it when you find it, and when you find your place in the yoga world and it could lead you to amazing things.

-Paula Peterson

THE PROBLEM

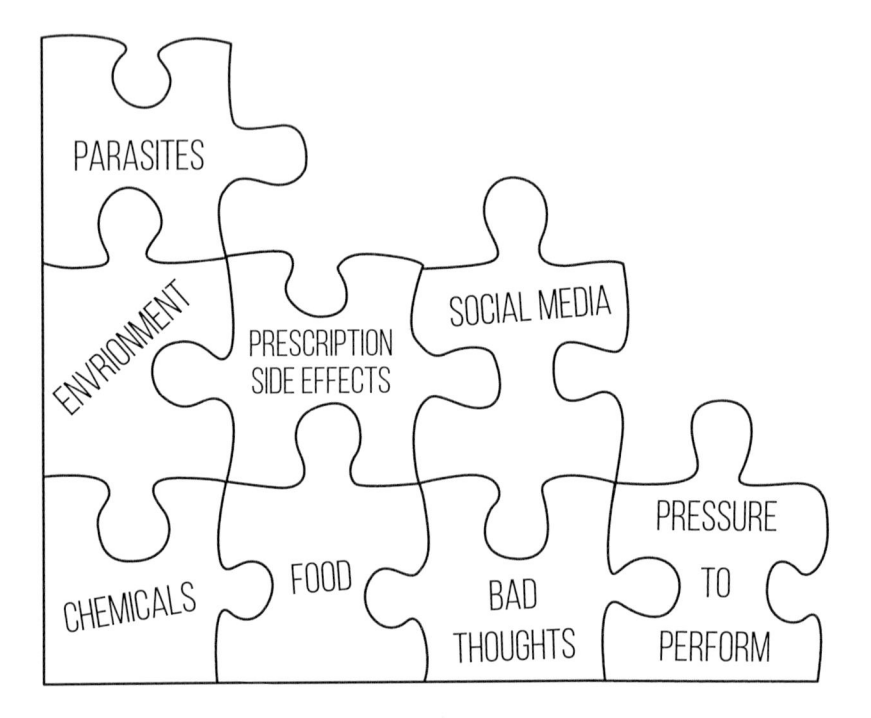

- PARASITES
- ENVRIONMENT
- PRESCRIPTION SIDE EFFECTS
- SOCIAL MEDIA
- CHEMICALS
- FOOD
- BAD THOUGHTS
- PRESSURE TO PERFORM

SOLVING THE PUZZLE OF ANXIETY

There are many individual pieces that can contribute to a diagnosis of anxiety. In the same way, the cure will likely be multifaceted.

THE SOLUTION

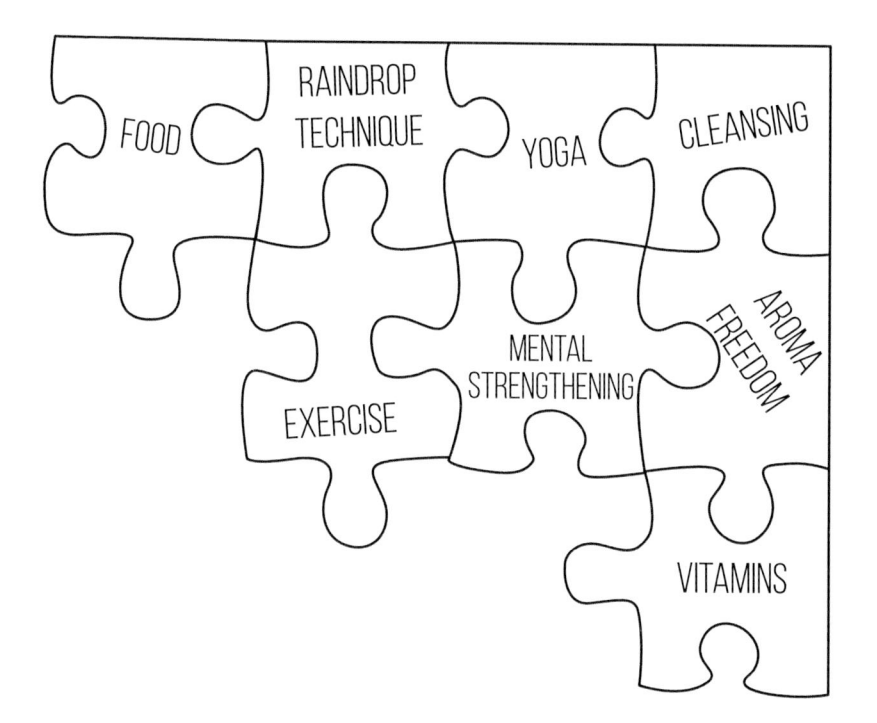

```
FOOD | RAINDROP TECHNIQUE | YOGA | CLEANSING
       EXERCISE | MENTAL STRENGTHENING | AROMA FREEDOM
                                         VITAMINS
```

It can be absolutely overwhelming to think of all the things that can contribute to poor mental health. That's why I recommend to start with just three things you can change today and move forward from there. Take a moment to set an intention for your personal journey and, when you're ready, flip over to the next page for a space to write down your thoughts.

PERSONAL REFLECTION

Accountability Journal

What are 3 things you can start doing today? What is your plan? What resonates with you?

1 _____

2 _____

3 _____

What are 3 toxic ingredients that you can cut back on?

1 _____

2 _____

3 _____

What are 3 things you can read or watch in the Resources section of this book?

1 _____

2 _____

3 _____

EPILOGUE

Be accountable to yourself. Be accountable to something. You have to want the change.

If you value your health, body, mind and spirit, then use some of this knowledge and be an advocate for yourself. There comes a time when you have to take responsibility for your choices. Stand up and boldly say, "I am the boss. I am in control. I am CHOOSING something better."

I chose to wake up and do something different.

If the results you're getting with your choices right now are serving you, and you are changing and growing in a positive direction, then keep doing what you're doing. But if you are stuck and in a downward spiral like I was, you have my permission to let go of what's not working and learn to try something new.

After years of being on this health journey and learning all I could about healing my family, I'm happy to say it was all worth it.

My Emily is now all grown up and happily married to an incredible man. She has two very healthy children, Noah and Leo, and she is an amazing mom. Even with two kids, I don't think I have seen anyone with so much patience! We love her sarcasm and sense of humor; she is always making the whole family laugh! Emily has such a big heart and loves helping others with problems she used to suffer from. She is smart. She loves to read and self-educate, and I am so proud of the woman she turned out to be.

My Samantha is a walking billboard for taking excellent care of herself and her daughter, Sophia. Her transformation has been incredible to watch. I watched her go from 50 pounds overweight, medicated and in emotional despair, to an energetic Pilates pro and role model. She is now guiding and leading a team of entrepreneurial women on their journey to better health.

My son Jonathan is also diving into natural remedies and takes excellent care of himself when it comes to food and exercise. He's even teaching me new things, from red light therapy to intermittent fasting! Never in my wildest dreams would I ever think this would happen. He is hardworking and so handsome. He's also 6'4" and single, if you're looking and in the market.

My husband Tom has seen a significant difference in his health while living a healthier lifestyle. He used to nap all the time, and he was always tired. Now, when he naps on occasion, it's completely different. He has energy like he did when we first started dating. We now have fewer health problems, less stress and a stronger relationship in our faith and marriage than ever before.

As for me, I have found an energy and passion I didn't know existed. My time is now spent helping people uncover the layers of what is holding them back. It's extremely rewarding and has changed me for a lifetime. I realized most of my stress was debt related because I don't have that problem anymore. I'll save that story for another book. I LOVE what I do and love being a witness to people's transformations! I actively share my story at speaking engagements and love inspiring others to think differently. This has now become the best ride our family has ever been on!

If you are overwhelmed, that is GOOD! That means you are considering trying a few things, and it's exactly where you want to be. If you've been inspired, I want you to cling to that emotion. Don't let it fade back into those limited beliefs that something like this can't happen for you too. Remember, I was exactly where you are right now: broke, sick and worn out from the stressors of the world.

So just start. Drink more water. Eat less sugar. Give just one supplement a chance for at least 90 days. Replace one chemical-laden product with a better one. Take a walk or get out that bike. Some of you will be overwhelmed and say screw it - others will say, "Bring it on, I'm ready." I'm talking to you.

Remember, it's all about the little things. It's all about how YOU are going to kick anxiety in the ass, a little at a time.

What will happen if you don't?

MY FAVORITE RESOURCES

BOOKS

- 25 to Life, by Adam Green
- Dangerous Beauty. The truth about cosmetics & personal care products, by Peter Dingle phD. Or purchase his book at www.drdingle.com
- Essentials: 75 Answers to Common Questions About Essential Oils, by Lindsey Elmore
- Feelings Buried Alive Never Die, by Karol Truman
- Guess What Came to Dinner?: Parasites & Your Health, by Ann Louise Gittleman
- Man Up, by Scott Schuler
- Mindful Breathing, Mindful Meditation & Mindful Kids Meditation Resources, by Pamela Hunter
- Releasing Emotional Patterns with Essential Oils, by Dr. Carolyn Mein
- The Aroma Freedom Technique: Using Essential oils to Transform Your Emotions and Realize Your Heart's Desire, by Benjamin Perkus
- The Four Year Career, by Richard Brooke
- The Obstacle is the Way: The Timeless Art of Turning Trials into Triumph, by Ryan Holiday

- The Total Money Makeover, by David Ramsey
- The Ultimate Introduction to NLP: How to Build a Successful Life, by Richard Bandler
- Vitamin Deficiency Symptoms & Cures: Modern Deficiency Illness - Using Intracellular Micronutrient Results - Vitamin Deficiencies can cause: diabetes, infertility, anxiety, fatigue, depression, by Dan Purser MD & Jared Larkin
- You are a Bad Ass, by Jen Sincero
- The Power of CBD & Essential Oils, by Dr. Oliver Wenker

DOCUMENTARIES

- Fed Up
- Food Inc.
- Sugar: The Bitter Truth
- That Sugar Film
- The Game Changers (available on Netflix)
- The Pharmacist
- What the Health
- Vaxxed

VIDEOS

- Quick Liver/Gallbladder Cleanse: You won't believe what your body can expel in one day. Don't be afraid.
- The 5 Second Rule by Mel Robbins
- The Cleansing Trio Video by Lindsey Elmore
- The Science of Thought, Caroline Leaf
- Laughter is the best medicine - You Tube

SHOP

- Full Script quality vitamins: I get my Magnesium from Orthomolecular.
- Oils and Beads: Aromatherapy bracelet kits
- Thrive Market: Wholesale organic foods
- Young Living: My life-changing purchase

WEBSITES/PEOPLE TO FOLLOW

- Center for Aromatherapy Research and Education (CARE): Raindrop Technique training and provider directory
- Environmental Working Group
- Food Babe: Investigating what's really in the food we eat
- Forever Young 2 Medical & Aesthetics Clinic: Carol Brinkman Hormone Specialist (Family Practice & Functional Medicine; she also tests for Parasites.)
- Gut Health Australia, Dr. Peter Dingle: Resource for real gut health
- Yoga with Adriene: A free yoga resource

OTHER

- Simply Being Phone App: Meditation guidance app
- Think Dirty App: A MUST-have.

CONTACT ME

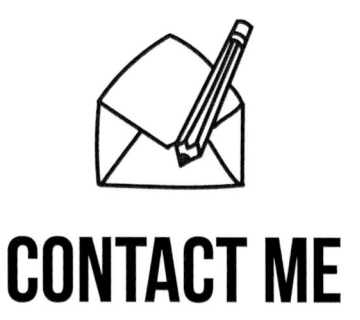

Website: www.stacytiegs.com

Email: stacy@stacytiegs.com

Join my Eat Real Food FaceBook Group

Join my Kicking Anxiety FaceBook Group

ACCOLADES

Thank you Jewels Whitehead for walking in my store with a bottle Joy™ Essential Oil.

Thank you to Dawn Meyer for showing me how to read labels and understand what real food is.

Thank you Scott and Brenda Shuler for being my inspiration and life coaches on this journey that I'm just getting started on.

Thank you to my entire family who listened to me for a very long time saying,

"I just need to finish my book".

A special thank you to my husband Tom Tiegs for always being so patient with me.

He makes our life easier in every way.

Thank you Justin Anderson from JiveMedia.co for showing me a better way in every aspect of my business. His inspiration, technical and business skills have empowered me to go kick ass no matter what. Justin and the Jive Media Team were phenomenal and guided me through this entire process. I highly recommend them!

Thank you Stacey Herman of www.so-connected.com for taking me through your Mental Strength Coaching Program and always supporting me. This has changed my life.

Thank you, Carol Brinkman for being my BFF and allowing me to have complete quiet and no distractions at your cabin to accomplish this goal.

Thank you Al Brinkman, Ed Daily and Pamela Hunter and Dr. Peter Dingle for being an incredible wealth of knowledge in my life.

Thank you to my amazing editor, Jen McCraw who pieced this all together for me and made this happen. Find her, you will love her. jenmccraw4@gmail.com

Thank you Paula Peterson and my entire team of friends for your love, encouragement and support.

Thank you Julie Senum for your wealth of knowledge, perspective and words of wisdom.

Thank you Lindsey Elmore for dialing up my branding and being a part of your Brand Strategies Lab that empowered me to think differently about who I am and what I'm about. I highly recommend this! Lindseyelmore.com/brandstrategieslab

Thank you Samantha Tiegs for polishing ALL my words, creating order, and giving this book your loving touch.

And thank you to all my friends who have worked with me back in the day and supported me through good times and bad. You all know who you are.

Yes, you. Definitely you.

ABOUT THE AUTHOR

Stacy Tiegs has been a small business owner and entrepreneur for over 15 years. Her passion is to educate and help people get to the root cause of their problems. She is a seeker of adventure and fun in everything she does. She's all about the little things that add up to the big things. Reading and studying natural health has made her a pillar in the natural health community. She is also certified in mental strength coaching and a professional from the old school of Hard Knocks.

ENDNOTES

1   Courtet, Philppe, and Jorge Lopez-Castroman. "Antidepressants and suicide risk in depression." World psychiatry : official journal of the World Psychiatric Association (WPA) vol. 16,3 (2017): 317-318. doi:10.1002/wps.20460.

2   What is a cell? (2017, May 17). Retrieved May 24, 2020, from https://www.yourgenome.org/facts/what-is-a-cell.

3   Gutierrez-Mazzotti, Claudia. "How Many Cells Do We Have in Our Body?" UCSB Science Line, UCSB Science Line, 12 Apr. 2013, scienceline.ucsb.edu/getkey.php?key=3926.

4   Nauert, Rick. "Liver Disorders Increase Risk of Depression and Anxiety in Young Adults." Psych Central, 8 Aug. 2018, psychcentral.com/news/2016/10/28/liver-disorders-increase-risk-of-depression-and-anxiety-in-young-adults/111763.html.

5   What is a GMO? (n.d.). Retrieved May 24, 2020, from https://www.nongmoproject.org/gmo-facts/what-is-gmo/.

6   Scheer, Roddy, and Doug Moss. "Dirt Poor: Have Fruits and Vegetables Become Less Nutritious?" Scientific American, 27 Apr. 2011, www.scientificamerican.com/article/soil-depletion-and-nutrition-loss/.

7   Wang, Xinhao, et al. "United States Drinking Water Quality Study Report." Uc.edu, Procter & Gamble Company, Dec. 2006, www.uc.edu/gissa/projects/drinkingwater/US_Drinking_Water_Quality_Project_report.pdf.

8   McCormack, Meredith. "Air Pollution." National Institute of Environmental Health Sciences, U.S. Department of Health and Human Services, www.niehs.nih.gov/health/topics/agents/air-pollution/index.cfm.

9   Shahroud University of Medical Sciences, et al. "The Effect of Chronic Exposure to Extremely Low-Frequency Electromagnetic Fields on Sleep Quality, Stress, Depression and Anxiety." Taylor & Francis, 29 Oct. 2018, www.tandfonline.com/doi/abs/10.1080/15368378.2018.154566

10   Admin. (2020, February 11). What is Blue Light? Retrieved May 24, 2020, from https://blutechlenses.com/blog/what-is-blue-light/.

11   Zhao, Zhi-Chun et al. "Research progress about the effect and prevention of blue light on eyes." International journal of ophthalmology vol. 11,12 1999-2003. 18 Dec. 2018, doi:10.18240/ijo.2018.12.20.

12   Madsen, Michael Tvilling et al. "The effect of MElatonin on Depressive symptoms, Anxiety, CIrcadian and Sleep disturbances in patients after acute coronary syndrome (MEDACIS): study protocol for a randomized controlled trial." Trials vol. 18,1 81. 23 Feb. 2017, doi:10.1186/s13063-017-1806-x.

13   "Social Media Anxiety Disorder." Social Media Anxiety Disorder - ETEC 510, 7 Feb. 2015, etec.ctlt.ubc.ca/510wiki/Social_Media_Anxiety_Disorder.

14   Kostoff, R., Heroux, P., Aschner, M., & Tsatsakis, A. (2020, January 25). Adverse health effects of 5G mobile networking technology under real-life conditions. Retrieved May 24, 2020, from https://www.sciencedirect.com/science/article/abs/pii/S037842742030028X?via=ihub.

15   Diamanti-Kandarakis, Evanthia, et al. "Endocrine-Disrupting Chemicals: an Endocrine Society Scientific Statement." Endocrine Reviews, The Endocrine Society, June 2009, www.ncbi.nlm.nih.gov/pmc/articles/PMC2726844/.

16   "Phthalates and DEHP." Health Care Without Harm, 31 Jan. 2020, noharm-uscanada.org/issues/us-canada/phthalates-and-dehp.

17   "Phthalates Factsheet." Centers for Disease Control and Prevention, 7 Apr. 2017, www.cdc.gov/biomonitoring/Phthalates_FactSheet.html.

18   O'Mahony, S.M., et al. "Serotonin, Tryptophan Metabolism and the Brain-Gut-Microbiome Axis." Behavioural Brain Research, Elsevier, 29 July 2014, www.sciencedirect.com/science/article/pii/S0166432814004768.

19   Steenbergen L, et al. "A Randomized Controlled Trial to Test the

Effect of Multispecies Probiotics on Cognitive Reactivity to Sad Mood." Brain, Behavior, and Immunity, U.S. National Library of Medicine, Aug. 2015, pubmed.ncbi.nlm.nih.gov/25862297-a-randomized-controlled-trial-to-test-the-effect-of-multispecies-probiotics-on-cognitive-reactivity-to-sad-mood/.

20 Reigstad CS, et al. "Gut Microbes Promote Colonic Serotonin Production Through an Effect of Short-Chain Fatty Acids on Enterochromaffin Cells." FASEB Journal : Official Publication of the Federation of American Societies for Experimental Biology, U.S. National Library of Medicine, Apr. 2015, pubmed.ncbi.nlm.nih.gov/25550456-gut-microbes-promote-colonic-serotonin-production-through-an-effect-of-short-chain-fatty-acids-on-enterochromaffin-cells/.

21 Reynolds, Tania A., et al. "Progesterone and Women's Anxiety across the Menstrual Cycle." Hormones and Behavior, Academic Press, 24 Apr. 2018, www.sciencedirect.com/science/article/abs/pii/S0018506X17303847.

22 https://www.ncbi.nlm.nih.gov/pmc/articles/PMC4457595/

23 Eske, J. (2019, August 21). Leaky gut syndrome: What it is, symptoms, and treatments. Retrieved May 24, 2020, from https://www.medicalnewstoday.com/articles/326117.

24 Jin, Mi-Joo et al. "The Relationship of Caffeine Intake with Depression, Anxiety, Stress, and Sleep in Korean Adolescents." Korean Journal of Family Medicine vol. 37,2 (2016): 111-6. doi:10.4082/kjfm.2016.37.2.111.

25 Lovallo, William R et al. "Caffeine stimulation of cortisol secretion across the waking hours in relation to caffeine intake levels." Psychosomatic Medicine vol. 67,5 (2005): 734-9. doi:10.1097/01.psy.0000181270.20036.06.

26 Wolde, Tsedeke. "Effects of Caffeine on Health and Nutrition: A Review." Research Gate, Food Science and Quality Management, 2014, www.researchgate.net/publication/279923885_Effects_of_caffeine_on_health_and_nutrition_A_Review.

27 Murphy, Michelle, and Julian G Mercer. "Diet-regulated anxiety." International Journal of Endocrinology vol. 2013 (2013): 701967. doi:10.1155/2013/701967.

28 Avena, Nicole M et al. "Evidence for sugar addiction: behavioral and neurochemical effects of intermittent, excessive sugar intake." Neuroscience and Biobehavioral Reviews vol. 32,1 (2008): 20-39. doi:10.1016/j.neubiorev.2007.04.019.

29 "How Much Sugar Do You Eat?" www.dhhs.nh.gov, New Hampshire Department of Health and Human Services, www.dhhs.nh.gov/dphs/nhp/documents/sugar.pdf.

30 "High-Fructose Diet in Adolescence May Exacerbate Depressive-like Behavior." Emory News Center, 19 Nov. 2014, news.emory.edu/stories/2014/11/fructose_adolescents_sfn/index.html.

31 Sharma, R P, and R A Coulombe. "Effects of Repeated Doses of Aspartame on Serotonin and Its Metabolite in Various Regions of the Mouse Brain." Food and Chemical Toxicology : an International Journal Published for the British Industrial Biological Research Association, U.S. National Library of Medicine, Aug. 1987, www.ncbi.nlm.nih.gov/pubmed/2442082.

32 Lindseth, Glenda N, et al. "Neurobehavioral Effects of Aspartame Consumption." Research in Nursing & Health, U.S. National Library of Medicine, June 2014, www.ncbi.nlm.nih.gov/pubmed/24700203/.

33 Ford, Rodney Philip Kinvig. "The Gluten Syndrome: A Neurological Disease." Medical Hypotheses, Churchill Livingstone, 29 Apr. 2009, www.sciencedirect.com/science/article/abs/pii/S0306987709002230?via=ihub.

34 Busby, Eleanor et al. "Mood Disorders and Gluten: It's Not All in Your Mind! A Systematic Review with Meta-Analysis." Nutrients vol. 10,11 1708. 8 Nov. 2018, doi:10.3390/nu10111708.

35 Chassaing, Benoit, et al. "Dietary Emulsifiers Directly Alter Human Microbiota Composition and Gene Expression Ex Vivo Potentiating Intestinal Inflammation." Gut, U.S. National Library of Medicine, Aug. 2017, www.ncbi.nlm.nih.gov/pubmed/28325746.

36 Noorafshan, Ali, et al. "Sodium Benzoate, a Food Preservative, Induces Anxiety and Motor Impairment in Rats.: Semantic Scholar." Semantic Scholar, Neurosciences, 1 Jan. 1970, www.semanticscholar.org/paper/Sodium-benzoate,-a-food-preservative,-induces-and-Noorafshan-Erfaniz adeh/7a3d67803db11fd7959bd8f45b1bcb215407ef1c.

37 Bateman, B, et al. "The Effects of a Double Blind, Placebo Controlled, Artificial Food Colourings and Benzoate Preservative Challenge on Hyperactivity in a General Population Sample of Preschool Children." Archives of Disease in Childhood, U.S. National Library of Medicine, June 2004, www.ncbi.nlm.nih.gov/pubmed/15155391.

38 Beezhold, Bonnie L, et al. "Sodium Benzoate-Rich Beverage Consumption Is Associated with Increased Reporting of ADHD Symptoms in College Students: a Pilot Investigation." Journal of Attention Disorders, U.S. National Library of Medicine, Apr. 2014, www.ncbi.nlm.nih.gov/pubmed/22538314.

39 Treatment, Center for Substance Abuse. "9 Substance-Induced Disorders." Substance Abuse Treatment for Persons With Co-Occurring Disorders., U.S. National Library of Medicine, 1 Jan. 1970, www.ncbi.nlm.nih.gov/books/NBK64178/.

40 Pleil, Kristen, et al. "Heavy Drinking Rewires Brain, Increasing Anxiety Problem." UNC Health Talk, 4 Sept. 2012, healthtalk.unchealthcare.org/heavy-drinking-rewires-brain-increasing-susceptibility-to-anxiety-problems/.

41 Victor, Maurice. "The Effects of Alcohol on the Nervous System." SpringerLink, Springer, Boston, MA, 1 Jan. 1992, link.springer.com/chapter/10.1007/978-1-4615-3320-7_14#citeas.

42 Vartanian, Lenny R et al. "Effects of soft drink consumption on nutrition and health: a systematic review and meta-analysis." American Journal of Public Health vol. 97,4 (2007): 667-75. doi:10.2105/AJPH.2005.083782.

43 Sánchez-Villegas, Almudena, et al. "Dietary Fat Intake and the Risk of Depression: The SUN Project." PLOS ONE, Public Library of Science, 26 Jan. 2011, journals.plos.org/plosone/article?id=10.1371/journal.pone.0016268.

44 Rao, T S Sathyanarayana et al. "Understanding nutrition, depression and mental illnesses." Indian Journal of Psychiatry vol. 50,2 (2008): 77-82. doi:10.4103/0019-5545.42391.

45 Miller, Michael M. "Low Sodium Chloride Intake in the Treatment of Insomnia and Tension States." Journal of the American Medical Association, American Medical Association, 22 Sept. 1945, jamanetwork.com/journals/jama/article-abstract/275931.

46 Heydarpour, F. "The Effect of Salt on Night Sleep." Endocrine Abstracts, 4 Dec. 2006, www.endocrine-abstracts.org/ea/0011/ea0011p590.

47 Kobylewski S and Jacobson, M. "Toxicology of Food Dyes." International Journal of Occupational and Environmental Health, U.S. National Library of Medicine, Sept. 2012, pubmed.ncbi.nlm.nih.gov/23026007-toxicology-of-food-dyes/.

48 Arnold, L Eugene et al. "Artificial food colors and attention-deficit/hyperactivity symptoms: conclusions to dye for." Neurotherapeutics: The Journal of the American Society for Experimental NeuroTherapeutics vol. 9,3 (2012): 599-609. doi:10.1007/s13311-012-0133-x.

49 Knouse, Laura E et al. "Depression in Adults with Attention-Deficit/Hyperactivity Disorder (ADHD): The Mediating Role of Cognitive-Behavioral Factors." Cognitive Therapy and Research vol. 37,6 (2013): 1220-1232. doi:10.1007/s10608-013-9569-5.

50 Hales, Craig, et al. "Prevalence of Obesity Among Adults and Youth: United States, 2015–2016." Centers for Disease Control, National Center for Health Statistics data brief, no 288. Hyattsville, MD: 2017, www.cdc.gov/nchs/data/databriefs/db288.pdf.

51 AL;, Lardner. "Neurobiological Effects of the Green Tea Constituent Theanine and Its Potential Role in the Treatment of Psychiatric and Neurodegenerative Disorders." Nutritional Neuroscience, U.S. National Library of Medicine, July 2014, pubmed.ncbi.nlm.nih.gov/23883567/.

52 Mao, Jun J, et al. "Long-Term Chamomile (Matricaria Chamomilla L.) Treatment for Generalized Anxiety Disorder: A Randomized Clinical Trial." Phytomedicine : International Journal of Phytotherapy and

Phytopharmacology, U.S. National Library of Medicine, 15 Dec. 2016, www.ncbi.nlm.nih.gov/pmc/articles/PMC5646235/.

53   AL;, Lardner. "Neurobiological Effects of the Green Tea Constituent Theanine and Its Potential Role in the Treatment of Psychiatric and Neurodegenerative Disorders." Nutritional Neuroscience, U.S. National Library of Medicine, July 2014, pubmed.ncbi.nlm.nih.gov/23883567/.

54   Gautam, Medhavi et al. "Role of antioxidants in generalised anxiety disorder and depression." Indian Journal of Psychiatry vol. 54,3 (2012): 244-7. doi:10.4103/0019-5545.102424.

55   Ganio, Matthew S., et al. "Mild Dehydration Impairs Cognitive Performance and Mood of Men: British Journal of Nutrition." Cambridge Core, Cambridge University Press, 7 June 2011, www.cambridge.org/core/journals/british-journal-of-nutrition/article/mild-dehydration-impairs-cognitive-performance-and-mood-of-men/3388AB36B8DF73E844C9AD19271A75BF.

56   Al Sunni, Ahmed, and Rabia Latif. "Effects of chocolate intake on Perceived Stress; a Controlled Clinical Study." International journal of health sciences vol. 8,4 (2014): 393-401.

57   Jackson, Sarah E., et al. "Is There a Relationship between Chocolate Consumption and Symptoms of Depression? A Cross-Sectional Survey of 13,626 US Adults." Wiley Online Library, John Wiley & Sons, Ltd, 29 July 2019, onlinelibrary.wiley.com/doi/abs/10.1002/da.22950.

58   Grases, G, et al. "Anxiety and Stress among Science Students. Study of Calcium and Magnesium Alterations." Magnesium Research, U.S. National Library of Medicine, June 2006, www.ncbi.nlm.nih.gov/pubmed/16955721

59   Kirkland, Anna E et al. "The Role of Magnesium in Neurological Disorders." Nutrients vol. 10,6 730. 6 Jun. 2018, doi:10.3390/nu10060730

60   Hilimire, Matthew R, et al. "Fermented Foods, Neuroticism, and Social Anxiety: An Interaction Model." Psychiatry Research, U.S. National Library of Medicine, 15 Aug. 2015, www.ncbi.nlm.nih.gov/pubmed/25998000.

61 Pullar, Juliet M et al. "High Vitamin C Status Is Associated with Elevated Mood in Male Tertiary Students." Antioxidants (Basel, Switzerland) vol. 7,7 91. 16 Jul. 2018, doi:10.3390/antiox7070091.

62 Kelley, L et al. "Vitamin D deficiency, behavioral atypicality, anxiety and depression in children with chromosome 22q11.2 deletion syndrome." Journal of developmental origins of health and disease vol. 7,6 (2016): 616-625. doi:10.1017/S2040174416000428.

63 Hidese, S., Ogawa, S., Ota, M., Ishida, I., Yasukawa, Z., Ozeki, M., & Kunugi, H. (2019). Effects of L-Theanine Administration on Stress-Related Symptoms and Cognitive Functions in Healthy Adults: A Randomized Controlled Trial. Nutrients, 11(10), 2362. https://doi.org/10.3390/nu11102362

64 Esmaily, H., Sahebkar, A., Iranshahi, M. et al. An investigation of the effects of curcumin on anxiety and depression in obese individuals: A randomized controlled trial. Chin. J. Integr. Med. 21, 332–338 (2015). https://doi.org/10.1007/s11655-015-2160-z.

65 Malcolm, Benjamin J, and Kimberly Tallian. "Essential oil of lavender in anxiety disorders: Ready for prime time?." The mental health clinician vol. 7,4 147-155. 26 Mar. 2018, doi:10.9740/mhc.2017.07.147.

66 Blessing, Esther M et al. "Cannabidiol as a Potential Treatment for Anxiety Disorders." Neurotherapeutics : the journal of the American Society for Experimental NeuroTherapeutics vol. 12,4 (2015): 825-36. doi:10.1007/s13311-015-0387-1.

67 "Exercise for Stress and Anxiety." Anxiety and Depression Association of America, ADAA, adaa.org/living-with-anxiety/managing-anxiety/exercise-stress-and-anxiety.

68 Geda, Yonas E, et al. "Engaging in Cognitive Activities, Aging, and Mild Cognitive Impairment: a Population-Based Study." The Journal of Neuropsychiatry and Clinical Neurosciences, U.S. National Library of Medicine, Apr. 2011, www.ncbi.nlm.nih.gov/pubmed/21677242.

69 Baxendale S, O'Sullivan J, Heaney D. Bright light therapy for symptoms of anxiety and depression in focal epilepsy: randomised controlled trial. Br J Psychiatry. 2013;202(5):352-356. doi:10.1192/bjp.bp.112.122119.

70 Shohani, Masoumeh et al. "The Effect of Yoga on Stress, Anxiety, and Depression in Women." International journal of preventive medicine vol. 9 21. 21 Feb. 2018, doi:10.4103/ijpvm.IJPVM_242_16.